INITIATING AND SUSTAINING THE
Clinical Nurse Leader Role

A Practical Guide

Edited by

JAMES L. HARRIS
DSN, RN, MBA, CNL, FAAN

Consultant
Washington, DC

LINDA ROUSSEL
DSN, RN, NEA-BC, CNL

Professor and Coordinator, Executive Nurse Administration Program
Clinical Nurse Leader Program
Mobile, Alabama

JONES AND BARTLETT PUBLISHERS
Sudbury, Massachusetts
BOSTON   TORONTO   LONDON   SINGAPORE

World Headquarters

Jones and Bartlett Publishers
40 Tall Pine Drive
Sudbury, MA 01776
978-443-5000
info@jbpub.com
www.jbpub.com

Jones and Bartlett Publishers
Canada
6339 Ormindale Way
Mississauga, Ontario L5V 1J2
Canada

Jones and Bartlett Publishers
International
Barb House, Barb Mews
London W6 7PA
United Kingdom

Jones and Bartlett's books and products are available through most bookstores and online booksellers. To contact Jones and Bartlett Publishers directly, call 800-832-0034, fax 978-443-8000, or visit our website, www.jbpub.com.

Substantial discounts on bulk quantities of Jones and Bartlett's publications are available to corporations, professional associations, and other qualified organizations. For details and specific discount information, contact the special sales department at Jones and Bartlett via the above contact information or send an email to specialsales@jbpub.com.

The authors, editor, and publisher have made every effort to provide accurate information. However, they are not responsible for errors, omissions, or for any outcomes related to the use of the contents of this book and take no responsibility for the use of the products and procedures described. Treatments and side effects described in this book may not be applicable to all people; likewise, some people may require a dose or experience a side effect that is not described herein. Drugs and medical devices are discussed that may have limited availability controlled by the Food and Drug Administration (FDA) for use only in a research study or clinical trial. Research, clinical practice, and government regulations often change the accepted standard in this field. When consideration is being given to use of any drug in the clinical setting, the health care provider or reader is responsible for determining FDA status of the drug, reading the package insert, and reviewing prescribing information for the most up-to-date recommendations on dose, precautions, and contraindications, and determining the appropriate usage for the product. This is especially important in the case of drugs that are new or seldom used.

Production Credits
Publisher: Kevin Sullivan
Acquisitions Editor: Emily Ekle
Acquisitions Editor: Amy Sibley
Associate Editor: Patricia Donnelly
Editorial Assistant: Rachel Shuster
Associate Production Editor: Katie Spiegel
Marketing Manager: Rebecca Wasley

V.P., Manufacturing and Inventory Control:
  Therese Connell
Composition: Forbes Mill Press
Cover Design: Scott Moden
Cover Image: © Worytko Pawel/ShutterStock, Inc.
Printing and Binding: Malloy, Inc.
Cover Printing: Malloy, Inc.

Library of Congress Cataloging-in-Publication Data
Harris, James L. (James Leonard), 1956-
  Initiating and sustaining the clinical nurse leader role : a practical guide / James L. Harris and Linda Roussel.
    p. ; cm.
  Includes bibliographical references and index.
  ISBN 978-0-7637-7631-2
  1. Nurse practitioners. 2. Nurse administrators. 3. Leadership. I. Roussel, Linda. II. Title.
  [DNLM: 1. Nurse Clinicians. 2. Leadership. 3. Nurse's Role. WY 128 H314i 2010]
  RT82.8.H37 2010
  610.7306'92—dc22
                            2009024155

6048
Printed in the United States of America
14 13 12 11 10   10 9 8 7 6 5 4 3 2

TABLE OF CONTENTS

CHAPTER EIGHT
Carol Boswell and Sharon Cannon

UNIT 6
ACADEMIC AND CLINICAL FOUNDATIONS FOR SUCCESSFUL CNL MATRICULATION

CHAPTER THIRTEEN

UNIT 7
**INITIATING AND SUSTAINING THE CLINICAL NURSE LEADER
ROLE: A PRACTICAL GUIDE**

CHAPTER SIXTEEN
James L. Harris

PREFACE

The constantly emerging and changing healthcare environment has spurred many discussions, forums, and summits over the past decade, culminating in a call to action. Stakeholders, consumers, and healthcare providers are leading a peaceful and staged revolution in nursing, known as the clinical nurse leader. Practice and education partnerships are forging forward with innovative strategies that are exponentially changing the direction of how care is delivered. Early adopters of the role have multiple outcomes that support how the role can transform care across a complete range of programs and services.

This textbook is a collection of innovative techniques and examples, provided by multiple academic and practice partners, that will be useful to clinical nurse leaders, students, and faculty, clinical partners, and administrators. We are grateful for the vision and courage of the membership of the American Association of Colleges of Nursing, Deans and Directors, the Department of Veterans Affairs, practice partners, clinical nurse leaders, and students who are matriculating through programs of study.

Thank you,
James L. Harris & Linda Roussel

ACKNOWLEDGMENTS

Support, focus, and innovation are hallmarks of great leaders. Such attributes capture the essence of the numerous individuals who envisioned a need for a new nursing role in response to the myriad of healthcare issues facing providers, administrators, and consumers of care. My colleague and trusted friend, Dr. Linda Roussel, and I are unable to identify each of the individuals who continuously direct energies and purposeful insight as the clinical nurse leader (CNL) role evolved. We acknowledge the insight of Dr. Geraldine "Polly" Bednash and Dr. Joan Stanley of the American Association of Colleges of Nursing (AACN), who through encouragement and support engaged nursing colleagues in thought and action as the CNL role was developed and implemented nationally. The efforts of the CNL Steering Committee, the current president and past presidents of the AACN, the AACN membership and board, and the AACN staff are recognized for their efforts and ongoing support for the CNL vision and the call to action to improve care for all Americans. The great vision and leadership by Ms. Cathy Rick, Chief Nursing Officer, Department of Veterans Affairs, to endorse the role and its implementation throughout Veterans Affairs is both visionary and central to quality care for America's heroes. Because of her efforts, CNLs are contributing to quality care and disseminating measureable outcomes nationally.

Both Linda and I would be remiss not to acknowledge the visionary foresight of Dr. Colleen Conway-Welch and Dr. Linda Norman from Vanderbilt University, and Dr. Debra Davis, Dr. Rosemary Rhodes, and Dr. Catherine Dearman from the University of South Alabama, who were early adopters and initiated CNL programs of study. Lastly, we acknowledge all faculty, students, and readers of the text.

James L. Harris

CONTRIBUTORS

Deborah Antai-Otong, MS, RN, CNS, NP, CS, FAAN
Veterans Integrated System Network
Arlington, TX

Bonnie B. Anton, MN, RN
University of Pittsburgh Medical Center
Pittsburgh, PA

Carol Boswell, EdD, RN, CNE, ANEF
Center of Excellence in Evidence-Based Practice
Texas Tech University Health Sciences Center
Odessa, TX

Stephanie S. Brown, MSN, RN, CNE
University of South Alabama Medical Center
Mobile, AL

Sharon Cannon, EdD, RN, ANEF
Center of Excellence in Evidence-Based Practice
Texas Tech University Health Sciences Center
Odessa, TX

Barbara M. Carranti, MS, RN, CNS
Le Moyne College
Syracuse, NY

Joan Shinkus Clark, MSN, RN, NEA-BC
SVP and Texas Health Chief
Arlington, TX

Debra C. Davis, DSN, RN
University of South Alabama College of Nursing
Mobile, AL

Catherine Dearman, PhD, RN
University of South Alabama College of Nursing
Mobile, AL

Elizabeth Furlong, PhD, JD, RN
Center for Health Policy and Ethics
Creighton University School of Nursing
Omaha, NE

Alice J. Godfrey, MPH, RN, BC
University of South Alabama College of Nursing
Mobile, AL

Christine Meyer, PhD, RN
McKesson Provider Technologies
Bridgeville, PA

Ramona Nelson, PhD, BC-RN, FAAN, ANEF
Slippery Rock University
R. Nelson Consulting
Allison Park, PA

Karen M. Ott, MSN, RN
Department of Veterans Affairs
Office of Nursing Services
Washington, DC

Joan M. Stanley, PhD, RN, CRNP, FAAN
American Association of Colleges of Nursing
Washington, DC

Patricia L. Thomas, PhD, RN, FACHE, CHE-BC, NEA-BC, ACNS-BC
University of Detroit–Mercy
Detroit, MI

Sandra E. Walters, DNP, RN
VA Tennessee Valley Healthcare System
Nashville, TN

Lonnie Williams, MSN, RN
New Orleans, LA

CNLs and CNL Students

Ellen M. Asbury, MS, BSN, RN
VAMHCS (Veterans Affairs Maryland Health Care System)
Baltimore, MD

Karen Bennett, BSN, RN, CNL
University of West Georgia
Carrollton, GA

Charlotte J. Birkenfeld, MSN, RN, CCRN, CNL
Malcom Randall Veterans Hospital
North Florida/South Georgia Veterans Health System
Gainesville, FL

Sally Brewer, RRT, NPS
Maine Medical Center
Portland, ME

Amanda Brown, MSN, RN, CNL, CPN
Wolfson Children's Hospital/Baptist Medical Center
Jacksonville, FL

Suzanne Brown, BSN, RN, CNL
University of West Georgia
Carrollton, GA

Michelle Carpentier, BSN, RN
The Miriam Hospital
Providence, RI

Micheline Chipman, MS, RN, CCRN
Maine Medical Center
Portland, ME

David Ciraculo, DO, MPH, FACS
Maine Medical Center
Portland, ME

Christine Cobb, MSN, RN
Malcom Randall Veterans Hospital
North Florida/South Georgia Veterans Health System
Gainesville, FL

Angela M. Creta, MS, RN, CNL
The Miriam Hospital
Providence, RI

Anjanetta Davis, MSN, RN, CNL
Springhill Medical Center
Mobile, AL

Janie Decker, BSN, RN, CNL
UMDNJ School of Nursing
Newark, NJ

Mary T. Dellario, MSN, RN, CNL
VAMHCS (Veterans Affairs Maryland Health Care System)
Baltimore, MD

Mary De Ritter, MSN, RN, CNL
Englewood Hospital and Medical Center
Englewood, NJ

Patricia Egan, MSN, RN, CNL
Sarasota County Health Department
Sarasota, FL

Kathy Faber, MSN, RN, CNL
St. Joseph's Regional Medial Center
Paterson, NJ

Jean Fecteau, MS, RN
Maine Medical Center
Portland, ME

Laurel Foster
Mease Dunedin Hospital
Dunedin, FL

Terri Gaiser, MSN, RN, CNL
Saginaw Valley State University
University Center, MI

Sara Gravelle, MSN, RN, CNL
Wolfson Children's Hospital/Baptist Medical Center
Jacksonville, FL

Kim Hall, MSN, RN, CNL
South Texas Veterans Health Care System
San Antonio, TX

Christina Hericks, MSN, RN, CNL
Cincinnati VAMC
Cincinnati, OH

Lisa Hubbard, MSN, RN, CNL, AHN-BC
Cincinnati VAMC
Cincinnati, OH

Jillian Jacob, MSN, RN, CNL
Cincinnati VAMC
Cincinnati, OH

Jennifer A. Jones, MSN, RN, CNL
Jersey City Medical Center
Jersey City, NJ

Shannon Kartchner, BSN, RN
George E. Wahlen Veterans Medical Center
Salt Lake City, UT

Diane L. Kelly, DrPH, MBA, RN, CNL
University of Utah
Salt Lake City, UT

Tammy Lee, MSN, RN, CNL
Springhill Medical Center
Mobile, AL

Mary Jo Loughlin, MSN, RN
Hunterdon Medical Center
Flemington, NJ

Lynne A. Ludeman, BS, RN, CNL(c)
Portland VA Medical Center
Portland, OR

Nicole Manchester, MSN, RN, CNL, CCRN
Maine Medical Center
Portland, ME

Lisa Maree, ARNP, CNL, CNS
North Florida/South Georgia Veterans Health System
Gainesville, FL

Mary E. Mather, MSN, RN
South Texas Veterans Health Care System
San Antonio, TX

Joel McMullin, BSRC, RRT
Maine Medical Center
Portland, ME

Robyn Mitchell, MSN, RN, CNL
VA Maryland Healthcare System
Baltimore, MD

Sonja Orff Ney, MS, RN, CNL
Maine Medical Center
Portland, ME

Rebecca Pomrenke, MSN, RN, CNL
University of South Alabama Medical Center
Mobile, AL

Darlene Rouleau, BSN, RN, CMS
Maine Medical Center
Portland, ME

Laurel B. Scaff, MS, RN, CNL
Mease Dunedin Hospital
Dunedin, FL

Connie Shipley, MS, BSN, RN, CNL
George E. Wahlen Department of Veterans Affairs Medical Center
Salt Lake City, UT

Jennifer Spiker, MS, RN, CNL
Portland VA Medical Center
Portland, OR

Mary Stachowiak, MSN, RN, CNL
Clinical Nurse Leader Association (CNLA)
Washington, DC

Judd E. Strauss, MSN, RN, CNL
Hunterdon Medical Center
Flemington, NJ

Dabuekke Tabor, MS, RN, CNL
Maine Medical Center
Portland, ME

Carrie Tierney, MSN, RN, CNL
South Texas Veterans Health Care System
San Antonio, TX

Suzanne VanBoening, RN-BC
Mary Lanning Memorial Hospital
Hastings, NE

Denise Walker, MSN, RN, CNL, CPON
Wolfson Children's Hospital/Baptist Medical Center
Jacksonville, FL

Sally Whitten, RRT
Maine Medical Center
Portland, ME

Unit 1
Introduction

ONE

Introducing the Clinical Nurse Leader: A Catalyst for Quality Care

■ Joan M. Stanley

Introduction

Health care is at a crossroads. Economic instability, mushrooming costs, rapid growth in biomedical advances, workforce shortages, changing population demographics, and demands for better outcomes all call for new ways of delivering health care and educating future health professionals. Nursing is faced with its own unique challenges, including the fragmentation of care, retention of nurses in the profession, opportunities for career advancement, utilization of nurses to the full scope of practice, and equipping clinicians with the knowledge and skills needed to address the competing demands of a complex healthcare system. Inter- and intraprofessional collaboration are key to meeting these challenges. Innovative partnerships between practice and education are even more critical in addressing and sustaining effective solutions for the long term. Within this healthcare environment, the American Association of

> "Imagination is the beginning of creation: you imagine that you desire, you will get what you imagine, and at last you create what you will."
>
> George Bernard Shaw

Colleges of Nursing (AACN), in partnership with practice leaders, has created the clinical nurse leader (CNL), the first new nursing role in over 40 years. The CNL is prepared to respond to today's challenges and readily adapt to meet the needs of the rapidly changing healthcare environment.

The Healthcare Environment

In 1999, the Institute of Medicine (IOM) released its landmark report, *To Err Is Human: Building a Safer Health System*, which estimated that up to 98,000 Americans die each year as a result of medical errors (IOM, 1999). Subsequent estimates indicated that these numbers may be even higher (Leape & Berwick, 2005). The estimated national costs of preventable adverse events (medical errors resulting in injury) are in the billions. In addition, medication-related errors and mistakes that do not result in actual harm are extremely costly and have a significant impact on the quality of care and healthcare outcomes. Over the past decade, the IOM and others, including the American Hospital Association (AHA), The Joint Commission, and the Robert Wood Johnson Foundation, have all called on healthcare systems to refocus their efforts to reduce medical errors, improve patient safety, and reevaluate how future health professionals will be educated (IOM, 2003; AHA Commission on Workforce for Hospitals and Health Systems, 2002; The Joint Commission, 2002; Kimball & O'Neil, 2002).

A report released by the AHA in 2007 estimated that U.S. hospitals needed approximately 116,000 registered nurses (RNs) to fill vacant positions nationwide. By 2020, federal officials with the Health Resources and Services Administration (HRSA) project that the nation's nursing shortage will intensify with more than 1 million new and replacement nurses needed. In addition by the year 2015, this shortage is projected to encompass the entire country, with all 50 states experiencing a shortage of nurses to varying degrees (Health Resources and Services Administration, 2006). The impact of the nursing shortage on the quality and outcomes of nursing care has dire consequences if not addressed. Needleman and associates demonstrated that lower nurse staffing levels were associated with adverse patient outcomes, including higher rates of pneumonia, urinary tract infections, length of stay, and "failure to rescue" (Needleman, Buerhaus, Mattke, Stewart, & Zelevinsky, 2002). Aiken and colleagues found that low nurse-to-patient ratios were related to higher risk-adjusted 30-day mortality and "failure to rescue" rates. In addition, nurses practicing in settings with lower nurse-to-patient ratios were more likely to experience burnout and job dissatisfaction (Aiken, Clarke, Sloane, Sochalski, & Silber, 2002).

In addition to the predictions for a long-lasting nursing shortage and the universal calls from outside nursing to change the way health professionals are educated and practice, several studies have demonstrated that more nurses educated at the baccalaureate levels or higher produced better patient outcomes, specifically reduced mortality and failure-to-rescue rates (Estabrooks, Midodzi, Cummings, Ricker, & Giovannetti, 2005; Aiken, Clarke, Cheung, Sloane, & Silber, 2003).

Leading the Profession to a New Vision for Nursing Education

In direct response to the changing global demographics, a healthcare system in turmoil, and drastic shortages of nursing professionals, the AACN has entertained an ongoing dialogue to examine and shape nursing education. For over a decade, this dialogue, including broad representation of stakeholders internal and external to nursing, focused on the knowledge, skills, and competencies needed by professional nurses to address the demands of an evolving healthcare system. From this dialogue has emerged a preferred future for nursing and new models for nursing education. This vision encompasses all levels of nursing education, from the baccalaureate degree to the doctorate (Stanley, 2008). The CNL, prepared at the master's degree level as an advanced generalist to practice in any healthcare setting, however, is the linchpin in this preferred future.

In 1999, the AACN Board of Directors formed the Task Force on Education and Regulation for Professional Nursing Practice (TFER). The task force developed new education models, including a model for the "new nurse" graduate, a clinician educated beyond the 4-year baccalaureate degree with a new license and legal scope of practice. After consultation with nurse executives, regulators, and other key stakeholders, the TFER determined that a new role was needed to differentiate professional nursing's scope of practice. At the same time, the National Council of State Boards of Nursing (NCSBN) indicated it was not possible to create a separate license for entry-level nurses educated at the associate and baccalaureate degree levels unless the roles were well differentiated.

In 2002, in response to the recommendations from the TFER, the AACN Board created TFER II, charged with examining what competencies were needed in the current and future healthcare system to improve patient care outcomes. A wide array of stakeholders, representing nursing education and practice, medicine, healthcare administration, pharmacy, public health, and others, were invited to provide input into what the "new nurse" role might look like. This work resulted in the 2003 publication of the *Working Paper on the Role of the Clinical Nurse Leader*. Prior to its publication, in addition to the competencies needed for this new role, many discussions were held within AACN and with external groups on a possible name for this new role and what educational preparation would be needed to prepare someone to practice at this level.

The CNL Initiative Is Born

Since these early stages in the evolution of this new role, the AACN Board has remained committed to the implementation of the CNL and the involvement of both education and practice. In 2003, the Implementation Task Force (ITF), comprised of representatives of both education and practice, was appointed to oversee the development of this new role. Modeling the importance of education-practice partnerships, the American Organization of Nurse Executives (AONE) was invited to appoint a representative to serve on the ITF. Another extremely important partner in this initiative has been the Department of Veterans Affairs (DVA). Cathy Rick, Chief Nursing Officer, as an early stakeholder, has been a proponent of the CNL from its early stages, and the DVA has participated at all levels in collaborating on the design and implementation of the CNL. This joint participation of education and practice has been a key factor in the success of the initiative. In January 2007, the ITF submitted its final report and recommendations to the AACN Board. Tremendous strides had been made in moving the CNL initiative forward; however, continued support and leadership by AACN was critical to sustaining the early momentum and ensuring continued growth. Responding to this recommendation, in March 2007, the AACN Board appointed the CNL Steering Committee, comprised also of education and practice representatives, whose primary charge was to elevate the visibility and sustainability of the CNL-advanced generalist role and measure the CNL's impact on patient care outcomes.

Key Steps and Landmarks Along the Way

In October 2003, AACN sent an open invitation to all deans of schools of nursing, inviting them to participate in an exploratory meeting on the CNL role, which included exploring the implications and expectations for education programs and the transformation of care delivery models. The only requirement of participants was that they attend with at least one nurse leader from a practice institution. Over 280 individuals representing 100 potential partnerships attended this exploratory meeting.

By March 2004, a request for proposal (RFP) was sent to all AACN member schools, inviting schools and their practice partners to commit to implementing the CNL role, including the design of master's-level CNL curriculum and integration of the CNL role within at least one unit in the practice setting. In June 2004, the ITF sponsored a CNL Implementation Conference for all education practice partners participating in the initiative. Representatives from 79 schools of nursing and 136 practice organizations participated, with the goal of advancing the CNL movement.

By fall 2006, the number of partnerships had grown to 87, representing 93 schools of nursing and 191 healthcare practice settings. The number has continued to grow and now includes 106 schools and over 200 practice settings.

Numerous forums and conferences, including annual CNL conferences, have been held since the initial CNL Implementation Conference in June 2004. Most recently, the joint AACN-DVA CNL Summit was held in New Orleans, Louisiana, in January 2009. Over 400 faculty members, deans, CNOs, CNLs, students, healthcare administrators, and physicians attended the summit, highlighting the success and growth of the CNL initiative. The newly created CNL Association (CNLA), open to all CNLs and students, held its inaugural meeting during the 2009 summit as well.

Another landmark decision was the development of a CNL certification examination and designation. CNL certification provides a unique credential for graduates of the master's and post-master's CNL programs. The CNL Certification Examination was piloted by 12 schools, November 2006–January 2007. The first regular administration of the CNL Certification Examination occurred in April–May 2007. Since that time over 600 CNLs have been certified and may use the credential and title CNL. The Commission on Nurse Certification (CNC) was formed in 2007. An elected board and staff oversee all certification related activities and policies.

AACN was also successful in trademarking the CNL title and the CNL Certification Examination in an effort to protect the integrity of this new designation. Only individuals who are successful in obtaining CNL certification may use the title CNL.

The CNL Role

The design of the CNL role was done in collaboration with constituents from a broad array of stakeholders within the healthcare system. As the role emerged, it became evident that many leaders in practice had already identified the need for a nurse with these skill and knowledge sets. Similar roles were being developed and emerging on an ad hoc basis in settings across the country. Nurses were being recruited to fill these roles based on availability, clinical experiences, and self-selection. In many instances these nurses were completing classroom and clinical experiences without receiving academic credit or recognition of the advanced competencies being acquired. In addition, there was no standardization of the competencies and experiences required, and the utilization of these nurses varied from site to site. All of these factors prevented these CNL forerunners from moving from one care setting to another, discouraged the duplication of care models, and made it difficult to assess the impact these clinicians were having on care outcomes.

Assumptions About the CNL

Ten assumptions about the CNL were made early on as role competencies were delineated and curricula designed. These assumptions included the following:

1. Practice is at the microsystem level.
2. Client care outcomes are the measure of quality practice.
3. Practice guidelines are based on evidence.
4. Client-centered practice is intra- and interdisciplinary.
5. Information will maximize self-care and client decision-making.
6. Nursing assessment is the basis for theory and knowledge development.
7. Good fiscal stewardship is a condition of quality care.
8. Social justice is an essential nursing value.
9. Communication technology will facilitate the continuity and comprehensiveness of care.
10. The CNL must assume guardianship for the nursing profession.[1]

Key Components of the CNL Role

The CNL is seen as a leader in the healthcare delivery system—not just the acute care setting, but in all settings in which health care is delivered. The implementation of

---

[1] Model C (see Table 1-1): Second-degree programs for individuals with a baccalaureate degree in another discipline are expected to prepare graduates with the CNL competencies in addition to the competencies delineated in the AACN (1998) *Essentials of Baccalaureate Education for Professional Nursing Practice.*

the CNL role, however, will vary across settings. The CNL is not an administrative or management role. The CNL assumes accountability for patient care outcomes through the assimilation and application of evidence-based information to design, implement, and evaluate patient plans of care. The CNL is a provider and manager of care at the point of care to individuals and cohorts of patients within a unit or healthcare setting. The CNL designs, implements, and evaluates patient care by coordinating, delegating, and supervising the care provided by the healthcare team, including licensed nurses, technicians, and other health professionals.

The defining aspects of CNL practice include the following:

- Leadership in the care of patients in and across all settings;
- Implementation of evidence-based practice in all healthcare settings for diverse and complex patients;
- Lateral integration of care for a specified group or cohort of patients;
- Clinical decision making;
- Design and implementation of plans of care;
- Risk anticipation, specifically evaluating anticipated risks to patient safety with the aim of quality improvement and preventing medical errors;
- Participation in identification and collection of care outcomes;
- Accountability for evaluation and improvement of point-of-care outcomes;
- Mass customization of care;
- Client and community advocacy;
- Education for individuals, families, groups, and other healthcare providers;
- Information management, including using information systems and technology at the point of care to improve healthcare outcomes;
- Delegation and oversight of care delivery and outcomes;
- Team leadership and collaboration with other health professional team members;
- Interprofessional communication;
- Leveraging human, environmental, and material resources;
- Management and use of client care and information technology; and
- Design and provision of health promotion and risk reduction services for diverse populations (AACN, 2007b).

An in-depth description of each of these practice components can be found in the AACN 2007 *White Paper on the Education and Role of the Clinical Nurse Leader* (AACN, 2007a).

Educating the CNL

As the CNL evolved, extensive dialogue occurred around the appropriate level of education to prepare someone to practice in this new role. Crosswalking the essential competencies for entry-level professional nurses with those identified for the advanced nurse generalist clearly showed that the additional knowledge, skills, and experiences needed to practice in this new role could not be obtained within a 4-year baccalaureate nursing program (AACN, 1998). Based on this evaluation and input from multiple stakeholders, the decision was made by the AACN board that the educational preparation of the CNL must be at the graduate level, in a master's or post-master's degree program.

In fall 2007, there were 1,270 students enrolled in 70 CNL programs, and in the 2006–2007 academic year, 265 students graduated from these CNL programs (Fang, Htut, & Bednash, 2008). By the following year, these numbers had grown to 1,650 students enrolled in 81 programs, with 467 graduates in the 2007–2008 academic year (Fang, Tracy, & Bednash, 2009). In addition, over 600 graduates of the CNL programs have been certified by CNC by this time.

The CNL Curriculum Framework

Assumptions about CNL graduate education programs include the following:

1. The education program culminates in a master's degree or post-master's degree in nursing.
2. The CNL graduate is prepared as an advanced generalist.
3. The CNL graduate will be competent to provide care at the point of care.
4. The CNL graduate will be prepared in clinical leadership for practice throughout the healthcare delivery system.
5. The CNL graduate is eligible to matriculate to a practice- or research-focused doctoral program.
6. The CNL graduate is prepared with advanced nursing knowledge and skills but does not meet the criteria for advanced practice registered nursing (APRN) scope of practice (APRN Consensus Work Group & National Council of State Boards of Nursing APRN Advisory Committee, 2008).
7. The CNL graduate is eligible to sit for the CNL Certification Examination.

The CNL Curriculum Framework encompasses three foci: nursing leadership, clinical outcomes management, and care environment management. Under each focus are major areas of emphasis, which are shown in Figure 1-1. Ten threads that should

Figure 1–1   CNL curriculum framework.

CNL CURRICULUM FRAMEWORK FOR CLIENT-CENTERED HEALTH CARE

Nursing Leadership

I.   Horizontal leadership
II.   Effective use of self
III.   Advocacy
IV.   Conceptual analysis of the CNL role
V.   Lateral integration of care

Clinical Outcomes Management

I.   Illness/disease management
 A.   Care management
 B.   Client outcomes
 C.   Builds on and expands the baccalaureate foundation in:
  1.   Pharmacology
  2.   Physiology/ pathophysiology
  3.   Health assessment
II.   Knowledge management
 A.   Epidemiology
 B.   Biostatistics
 C.   Measurement of client outcomes
III.   Health promotion and disease reduction/prevention management
 A.   Risk assessment
 B.   Health literacy
 C.   Health education and counseling
IV.   Evidence-based practice
 A.   Clinical decision making
 B.   Critical thinking
 C.   Problem identification
 D.   Outcome measurement

Care Environment Management

I.   Team coordination
 A.   Delegation
 B.   Supervision
 C.   Interdisciplinary care
 D.   Group process
 E.   Handling difficult people
 F.   Conflict resolution
II.   Healthcare finance/economics
 A.   Medicare and Medicaid reimbursement
 B.   Resource allocation
 C.   Healthcare technologies
 D.   Healthcare finance and socioeconomic principles
III.   Healthcare systems and organizations
 A.   Unit-level health care
 B.   Delivery/microsystems of care
 C.   Complexity theory
 D.   Managing change theories
IV.   Healthcare policy
V.   Quality management/risk reduction/patient safety
VI.   Informatics

Major Threads Integrated Throughout Curriculum

I.   Critical thinking/clinical decision making
II.   Communication
III.   Ethics
IV.   Human diversity/cultural competence
V.   Global health care
VI.   Professional development in the CNL role
VII.   Accountability
VIII.   Assessment
IX.   Nursing technology and resource management
X.   Professional values, including social justice

Source: AACN. (2007). *White Paper on the Education and Role of the Clinical Nurse Leader,* p. 32.

Table 1-1   CNL Curriculum Models

Model	Program Description
Model A	Program designed for BSN graduates
Model B	Program designed for BSN graduates; includes a post-BSN residency that awards master's credit toward the CNL degree
Model C	Program for individuals with a baccalaureate degree in another discipline; also known as a second-degree or generic master's
Model D	Program designed for ADN graduates; also known as an RN-MSN program
Model E	Post-master's certificate program

be integrated throughout the curriculum in didactic and clinical experiences are also identified. The actual design of the curriculum rests with the faculty at the schools of nursing. However, the expectation is that the graduate will be prepared with the competencies delineated in the AACN *White Paper* as well as the required clinical experiences (AACN, 2007a). The immersion experience is a critical component of the CNL curriculum. In addition to other clinical experiences integrated throughout the program, the immersion includes a minimum of 300 hours in practice in the CNL role with a designated clinical preceptor and a faculty partner. Many education programs in partnership with a clinical practice site designate a single preceptor but also involve a variety of other individuals—for example, someone from human resources, a financial officer, a quality improvement officer, a patient safety officer, and a nursing educator—in the preceptorship of the CNL student.

CNL Curricular Models

Five curricular models for graduate CNL education programs have emerged. These five models are shown in Table 1-1. The percentage of schools that have implemented each type of model are shown in Figure 1-2.

Where CNLs Are Practicing

The CNL competencies delineated in the *White Paper* prepare the nurse to practice as a leader in any healthcare setting (AACN, 2007a). Stakeholders who were asked

Figure 1-2   Percentage of schools offering CNL curriculum models (n = 99).

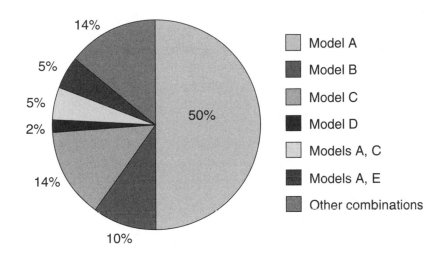

CNL EDUCATION MODELS.

14%
5%
5%
2%
14%
10%
50%

- Model A
- Model B
- Model C
- Model D
- Models A, C
- Models A, E
- Other combinations

Source: AACN CNL database 03/09.

to review early documents describing the CNL role and competencies unanimously stated that the nurse prepared with this set of competencies would be a valuable asset to their area of nursing practice or practice setting. The implementation of the CNL, however, does vary across settings, and the CNL's day-to-day activities will differ depending upon the setting, patient population, and care delivery model. To be most successful in any setting, however, the care delivery should be reshaped and the CNL integrated into this revised model to fully use the unique skill and knowledge set brought to the point of care by this new nurse.

CNLs are practicing and making a significant impact in a variety of practice sites. A majority of the early graduates are practicing in acute care hospitals where demands for improved outcomes and better ways of delivering care have been well documented. However, CNLs are migrating to other employment settings including school health, long-term care, outpatient clinics, home care, emergency departments, and state health departments. The employment settings for the early certified CNLs are shown in Table 1-2.

Table 1-2   Employment Sites for Certified CNLs

CNL(r) Employment Settings (*N* = 535)

Acute care inpatient	304
Community/public health	11
Home health	6
School/university health	24
Nursing home/long-term care/subacute care	7
Hospice	1
Hospital outpatient	7
Outpatient clinic/or surgery center	22
Physician practice	2
Nurse-managed practice	2
School of nursing	89
Other	60

Source: CNC certification database 3/09.

Impact of the CNL Role on Care Outcomes

As the number of CNLs in practice increases, the impact on patient care outcomes is becoming apparent. Much of the impact and cost benefits being reported are anecdotal. However, the outcomes being reported in lay and professional publications and at professional conferences are increasing rapidly. Stanley et al. reported outcomes of care at three healthcare settings located in one state (Stanley et al., 2008). These outcomes included improvement in the Centers for Medicare & Medicaid Services (CMS) core measures, for example, pain management, acute myocardial infarction (AMI), congestive heart failure (CHF), and pneumonia indicators; improved care coordination; improved physician-nurse collaboration; improved patient satisfaction; and decreased nurse turnover.

Gabuat et al. reported on a CNL pilot initiative that was conducted on a progressive care unit and medical/surgical unit at a for-profit hospital. Initially designed to be budget neutral, outcomes pre- and post-CNL implementation on these units also included decreased nursing turnover, increased patient and physician satisfaction, and improved core measures (acute MI, CHF, and pneumonia; Gabuat, Hilton, Kinnaird, & Sherman, 2008). Hartranft, Garcia, and Adams (2007) reported significant patient safety improvements that included zero falls with injury and nosocomial infections and pressure ulcers, improved patient satisfaction, and 100% achievement of CMS core measures after implementation of the CNL role on several units. In addition, Hartranft notes that many of the outcomes achieved by the CNL are not captured in hard data. For that reason the CNLs at this facility keep a daily journal of "saves" and qualitative accomplishments, for example, identifying the need for early intervention and ability to stabilize a patient without moving to a higher level of care (a savings of approximately $1,150 per day just for the bed; p. 263). Other identified outcomes have been the improvement in goal setting, greater engagement of staff nurses in projects, and improved nurse and physician satisfaction.

The Department of Veteran Affairs (DVA) has been involved in the early implementation of the CNL role, and the Veterans Health Administration is moving to fully implement the CNL role across all VA settings by the year 2016 (Verbal communication from James L. Harris). One of the first VA settings in which the CNL role was implemented was the Tennessee Valley Health Care System (TVHS). AACN and TVHS collaborated on a pilot of an evaluation tool to capture clinical outcomes pre- and postassignment of unit-based CNLs (Harris, Walters, Quinn, Stanley, & McGuinn, 2006). Preliminary findings from this pilot were positive and encouraging, including decreased readmission rates for patients discharged with CHF; decreased length of stay for patients with CHF; increased discharge instructions for patients with CHF on an acute medical unit; and decreased patient falls and surgical infection rates 30 days postoperative on an acute surgical unit. Since these early outcomes were reported, evaluation has been ongoing at TVHS, and the outcomes on five care units (microsystems of care) were recently reported. Significant outcomes were demonstrated, including a 20% decrease in patients receiving a blood transfusion posttotal knee arthroplasty (TKA) on a surgical inpatient unit, a 28.6% increase in venous thromboembolism prophylaxis implementation for critically ill intubated patients, and an 8% increase in participation in a restorative dining program on a transitional care unit (Hix, McKeon, & Walters, 2009).

Other reported outcomes linked to CNL practice include an 18.2% decrease in critical care days and a 40% decrease in returns to the critical care unit, netting an $800,000 savings over a 14-month period after a CNL implemented multidisciplinary rounds on long-term ventilator patients. Another CNL collaborated with a team of orthopedic surgeons and blood bank personnel to evaluate and then eliminate retransfusion of blood cells in TKA patients, which led to decreased opportunities for infection and netted an estimated $100,000 savings in time and equipment. At another facility, a CNL was able to decrease peripheral inserted central catheter (PICC) line infections from 179 blood stream infections (40 were related to the PICC line) to zero infections, netting an estimated $500,000 savings over a 12-month period (Wiggins, 2008). These projects and their impact on patient safety and quality of care do not represent the entire impact that these three CNLs made in that particular setting. Rather, they represent three documented examples of the impact the CNL has had in just three care settings. Increasingly, positive outcomes on quality of care and the related cost benefits are being reported by healthcare settings in which the CNL has been implemented. Although most of these examples are from acute care units, similar benefits and outcomes are being reported from a variety of care settings.

Future of CNL Education and Role

Although the CNL is not the sole answer to the many issues that plague the healthcare delivery system, it is one very promising strategy that is demonstrating a significant and sustained impact across settings. Calls for major changes in the way health care is delivered and the way health professionals are educated have prompted nursing education and practice, under AACN's leadership, to develop a preferred vision for nursing education with the CNL at the center. The CNL, an advanced generalist, is not a replacement for nurses in other roles, such as the clinical nurse specialist, nurse practitioner, nurse manager, or the staff nurse. Rather, the CNL is complementary to nurses in other roles who work in tandem with these providers to deliver high quality, patient-centered nursing care (Spross, Hamric, Hall, Minarik, Sparacino, & Stanley, 2004; Ott & Haase-Herrick, 2006). Healthcare leaders have identified the CNL as the future leader of quality improvement in the microsystem and at the point of care. The CNL initiative complements other quality improvement initiatives underway, such as the Robert Wood Johnson Foundation's (RWJF) Transforming Care at the Bedside (TCAB), which also has greatly impacted the quality of care available in hospitals (Robert Wood Johnson Foundation, 2008). CNLs in a number of settings are taking a lead in TCAB sites to implement quality improvement projects and improve patient safety. Partnering between education and practice has been identified as critical; collaboration and combining efforts are also crucial to making a lasting impact on enhancing care delivery.

The CNL initiative has grown considerably in the 5 years since the publication of the AACN *Working Paper*, which is now the *White Paper on the Education and Role of the Clinical Nurse Leader* (AACN, 2007a). The number of schools implementing CNL master's or post-master's programs has increased rapidly, and more schools are exploring the possibility of launching an advanced generalist program. For a number of schools, the CNL master's program represents the first graduate program offered at that institution. For others, the CNL master's program is an evolution as advanced specialty nursing programs are transitioned to the Doctor of Nursing Practice (DNP) degree. The number and type of healthcare institutions partnering with schools to implement the CNL has also expanded. As the impact of the CNL on patient safety, quality care outcomes, and cost benefits is more widely disseminated, it is anticipated that this expansion will occur exponentially. Particularly in this era of healthcare reform, cost containment, and changing reimbursement policies, the integration of the CNL into care delivery across settings offers a positive means of addressing these system-wide priorities.

AACN remains steadfast in its support for the CNL initiative. However, to sustain the momentum and assure that CNL becomes embedded within the healthcare delivery infrastructure, ongoing networking and expansion of national to local partnerships are critical. Documentation and broad dissemination of the CNL impact on patient safety, quality improvement, and the related cost benefits across a variety of healthcare settings also will be vitally important to sustaining this movement and embracing the CNL as a catalyst for quality care.

References

AHA Commission on Workforce for Hospitals and Health Systems. (2002). *In our hands: How hospital leaders can build a thriving workforce.* Chicago: American Hospital Association.

Aiken, L. H., Clarke, S. P., Cheung, R. B., Sloane, D. M., & Silber, J. H. (2003). Educational levels of hospital nurses and surgical patient mortality. *Journal of the American Medical Association, 290*(12), 1617–1623.

Aiken, L. H., Clarke, S. P., Sloane, D. M., Sochalski, J., & Silber, J. H. (2002). Hospital nurse staffing and patient mortality, nurse burnout, and job dissatisfaction. *Journal of the American Medical Association, 288*(16), 1987–1993.

American Association of Colleges of Nursing (AACN). (1998). *The essentials of baccalaureate education for professional nursing practice.* Washington, DC: Author.

American Association of Colleges of Nursing (AACN). (2007a). *White paper on the education and role of the clinical nurse leader.* Washington, DC: Author, pp. 6–10. Available at http://www.aacn.nche.edu/Publications/WhitePapers/ClinicalNurseLeader07.pdf

American Association of Colleges of Nursing (AACN). (2007b). *White paper on the education and role of the clinical nurse leader.* Washington, DC: Author, pp. 10–11. Available at http://www.aacn.nche.edu/Publications/WhitePapers/ClinicalNurseLeader07.pdf

APRN Consensus Work Group & National Council of State Boards of Nursing APRN Advisory Committee. (2008). *Consensus model for APRN regulation: Licensure, accreditation, certification & education*. Available at http://www.aacn.nche.edu/Education/pdf/APRNReport.pdf

Estabrooks, C. A,, Midodzi, W. K., Cummings, G. C., Ricker, K. L., & Giovannetti, P. (2005). The impact of hospital nursing characteristics on 30-day mortality. *Nursing Research, 54*(2), 74–84.

Fang, D., Htut, A. M., & Bednash, G. D. (2008). *2007–2008 enrollment and graduations in baccalaureate and graduate programs in nursing*. Washington, DC: American Association of Colleges of Nursing.

Fang, D., Tracy, C., & Bednash, G. D. (2009). *2008–2009 enrollment and graduations in baccalaureate and graduate programs in nursing*. Washington, DC: American Association of Colleges of Nursing.

Gabuat, J., Hilton, N., Kinnaird, L. S., & Sherman, R. O. (2008). Implementing the clinical nurse leader role in a for-profit environment. *Journal of Nursing Administration 38*(6), 302–307.

Harris, J. L., Walters, S. E., Quinn, C., Stanley, J., & McGuinn, K. (2006). *The clinical nurse leader role: A pilot evaluation by an early adopter*. Available at http://www.aacn.nche.edu/CNL/pdf/tk/VAEvalSynopsis.pdf

Hartranft, S. R., Garcia, T., & Adams, N. (2007). Realizing the anticipated effects of the clinical nurse leader. *Journal of Nursing Administration, 37*(6), 261–263.

Health Resources and Services Administration. (2006). *What is behind HRSA's projected supply, demand, and shortage of registered nurses?* Retrieved March 6, 2009, from http://bhpr.hrsa.gov/healthworkforce/reports/behindrnprojections/index.htm

Hix, C., McKeon, L., & Walters, S. (2009). Clinical nurse leader impact on clinical microsystems outcomes. *Journal of Nursing Administration, 39*(2), 71–76.

Institute of Medicine (IOM). (1999). *To err is human: Building a safer health system*. Washington, DC: National Academy Press, p. 1.

Institute of Medicine (IOM). (2003). *Health professions education: A bridge to quality*. Washington, DC: National Academies Press.

The Joint Commission. (2002). *Health care at the crossroads, strategies for addressing the evolving nursing crisis*. Chicago: Author.

Kimball, B., & O'Neil, E. (2002). *Health care's human crisis: The American nursing shortage*. Princeton, NJ: The Robert Wood Johnson Foundation.

Leape, L. L., & Berwick, D. M. (2005). Five years after to err is human. *Journal of the American Medical Association, 293*(19), 2384–2390.

Needleman, J., Buerhaus, P., Mattke, S., Stewart, M., & Zelevinsky, K. (2002, May 30). Nurse-staffing levels and the quality of care in hospitals. *New England Journal of Medicine, 346*(22), 1715–1722.

Ott, K. M., & Haase-Herrick, K. (2006). *Working statement comparing the clinical nurse leader and nurse manager roles: Similarities, differences and complementarities*. Washington, DC: AACN. Available at http://www.aacn.nche.edu/CNL/pdf/tk/roles3-06.pdf

Robert Wood Johnson Foundation. (2008). *The Transforming Care at the Bedside (TCAB) toolkit.* Retrieved March 5, 2009, from http://www.rwjf.org/qualityequality/product.jsp?id=30051

Spross, J. A., Hamric, A. B., Hall, G., Minarik, P. A., Sparacino, P. A., & Stanley, J. M. (2004). *Working statement comparing the clinical nurse leader and clinical nurse specialist roles: Similarities, differences and complementarities.* Washington, DC: AACN. Available at http://www.aacn.nche.edu/CNL/pdf/CNLCNSComparisonTable.pdf

Stanley, J. M. (2008). AACN shaping a future vision for nursing education. In B. A. Moyer and R. A. Wittmann-Price (Eds.), *Nursing Education: Foundations for Practice Excellence* (pp. 299–311). Philadelphia: F. A. Davis.

Stanley, J. M., Gannon, J., Gabuat, J., Hartranft, S., Adams, N., Mayes, C., et al. (2008). The clinical nurse leader: A catalyst for improving quality and patient safety. *Journal of Nursing Management, 16(5)*, 614–622.

Verbal communication from James L. Harris, Deputy Chief Nursing Officer, Department of Veterans Affairs, March 6, 2009.

Wiggins, M. (2008). *The clinical nurse leader demands in healthcare require new innovation.* Presentation made to The Joint Commission–Nursing Advisory Council, June 8, 2008, Oakbrook, IL.

Unit 2
Academic, Clinical, and Community Partnerships

TWO

Creating and Maintaining Academic, Clinical, and Community Partnerships

■ **Sandra E. Walters**

■ Learning Objectives

- ■ Identify the significance of partnerships in the implementation of the CNL role.
- ■ Identify core values for the CNL in developing and sustaining partnerships.
- ■ Identify core competencies needed for the CNL to support partnerships.
- ■ Define partnerships.
- ■ Describe the steps requisite to creating academic, clinical, and community partnerships.
- ■ Identify exemplars of partnerships in the implementation of the CNL role.
- ■ Describe the process for sustaining academic, clinical, and community partnerships.

> "There is no peace among equals because equality doesn't exist in this universe. Either one prevails or the other follows, or both negotiate their differences and create a greater partnership."
>
> Harold J. Duarte-Bernhardt

Key Terms

Partnership   Altruism
Accountability   Integrity
Needs assessment

CNL Roles

Client and community advocate   Coordinator of client care
Cultivator of partnerships with   Manager of care
   patients, families, groups, and   Effective communicator
   communities   Interpreter and user of qualitative data

CNL Professional Values

Altruism   Integrity
Accountability

CNL Core Competencies

Communication   Nursing technology and resource
Critical thinking   management

Introduction

A shortage of nurses in the United States focused the attention of clinicians, academicians, and communities on its causes, impacts, and possible solutions. The results of multiple studies have included recommendations for the development of academic and clinical relationships as partnerships between organizations. As early as 1998, the Pew Health Professions Commission called for the development of partnerships for the education of health professionals that would integrate the commitments of the care delivery systems with those of health education professionals and the needs of the communities served. In similar manner, a study by the Institute of Medicine (2000) resulted in recommendations for increased collaboration between institutions as a means to enhance patient safety, and the Robert Wood Johnson Foundation called for new practice models to enhance education-practice partnerships (Kimball & O'Neil, 2002). Additionally, the National League for Nursing (2003) called for nurse educators, students, consumers, and nursing service representatives to form partnerships that would dramatically reform learning and teaching, and would enhance the relationships between and among students, teachers, researchers, and clinicians.

Efforts to address the need to transform professional nursing care and nursing education led to the development of four separate task forces by American Association of Colleges of Nursing (AACN). With the establishment of an implementation task force to launch the clinical nurse leader role through education-practice partnerships, AACN ushered in an educational model that would be responsive to the changing needs of the healthcare environment (AACN, 2007a). The development of partnerships between educators, clinicians, and communities is an essential element to the successful implementation of the CNL role and forms the foundation for education and practice.

Partnership

The word *partnership* was derived in the 14th century from the Middle English use of the word *partner*. The original meaning was one that designated joint heirs or part holders and was itself derived from the Anglo-French word *parcener*, which referred to a division or share (*Merriam-Webster Online Dictionary*, 2008). Terms that appear closely related to the concept of partnership include *partner*, *partnering*, *part*, *partnered*, *partial*, and *partition*. These words have also evolved from the word *partner* and are generally used to describe a relationship in which there is a division or sharing of some larger whole with joint rights or responsibilities. The use of the term *partnership* appears in many forms, including those used to describe legal transactions as may be seen in a business, personal relationships that may express the state of committed bonding between two individuals, and even as a way of describing individuals who engage in a specific activity together, such as dancing.

A *partnership* can be defined as an alliance or union between individuals or groups that is characterized by mutual cooperation and responsibility to achieve a specified goal (*American Heritage College Dictionary*, 2007). Gallant, Beaulieu, and Carnevale (2002) and Hook (2006) focused on the context of the professional-patient relationship in partnerships. Their work established attributes for partnership

"Friendship is essentially a partnership."

Aristotle

such as shared decision making, relationships, professional competence, shared knowledge, autonomy, communication, participation, and shared power. Steinhart and Alsup (2001) identified trust, effective communications, shared values, monitoring programs, and long-term relationships as necessary in the formation of successful partnerships. In similar manner, the European Foundation for Quality Management (EFQM) model for health care includes partnership development as one of the eight elements of quality improvement (Vallejo et al., 2006). Their content analysis included the following elements of their model on partnership as:

- Requiring clearly identified mutual benefit;
- Consisting of shared goals;
- Being supported with expertise, resources, and knowledge;
- Delivering enhanced value to stakeholders by optimizing core competencies; and
- Building a sustainable relationship based on trust, respect, and openness.

Creating Academic, Clinical, and Community Partnerships

Antecedents for development of partnership within the CNL role must include recognition of unmet needs within the partner settings. In the education arena, unmet needs arise as the result of factors such as faculty vacancies, space constraints, limited equipment or supply resources, increased population diversity, and a lack of available practice models (Stanley, Hoiting, Burton, Harris, & Norman, 2007; Stark, 2003).

In the clinical arena unmet needs may result from increased complexity of the healthcare environment, the rapid advances in technology, an aging population, or licensure and certification requirements to maintain a well-educated, professional work force (Bartels, 2005; Bartels & Bednash, 2005; Zahner & Gredig, 2005). A review of hospital initiatives to support the education of nurses cited drivers for the formation of partnerships as including the need for: mechanisms whereby nurses could balance work and education, mechanisms for delivery of continuing education, the need for increased levels of nurses with BSN and MSN degrees, and pressures to decrease recruitment and retention costs (Cheung & Aiken, 2006).

Box 2-1   Gap Analysis

1. Determine the current state of the organization or microsystem in terms of available resources, performance, goals, values, knowledge, or internal and external constraints using performance data, stakeholder input, employee responses, or other sources.
2. Determine the desired or necessary state based on stakeholder input, benchmark data, community standards, or other comparison measures.
3. Analyze the gap between the current and desired states to identify problems, opportunities, strengths, weaknesses, or other concerns.
4. Prioritize needs and determine their importance to meeting organizational objectives, cost effectiveness, impact on stakeholders, or other goals.
5. Identify potential solutions and opportunities for improvements.

In communities, in addition to their roles as employers and procurers of goods and services, clinical and education partners may be needed to produce additional benefits, including being a source of volunteers, positively affecting productivity and safety, and acting as a source of health promotion. Concurrently, communities can contribute to health care through the provision of expertise as demonstrated by enterprises such as the auto industry, whose human factors engineering has been applied to health care (Kerfoot, Rapala, Ebright, & Rogers, 2006).

When unmet needs are recognized within the academic, clinical, and community institutions, the evaluation of the suitability of partnership may then progress. The role of the CNL in the formation of partnerships at any level should begin with a needs assessment or gap analysis. This systematic collection of information will be necessary for setting goals, developing an implementation plan, allocating resources, and establishing success indicators (See Box 2-1).

In order for a partnership relationship to be formed, the essential attributes of trust, respect, openness, and shared values must be present within the proposed relationship. If any of these is absent, the partnership will fail to progress and needs will continue to be unmet. If the essential attributes are present, however, the partnership will progress with the formulation of shared goals, establishment of communication strategies, designation of resources to be shared, and the designation of a monitoring program (Gallant et al., 2002).

The role of the CNL as a facilitator in the establishment of partnerships provides the opportunity to implement strategies to ensure the success of the initiatives. From the beginning, sharing of information with stakeholders throughout all involved organizations is crucial to successful implementation of partner initiatives. The clinical, academic, and community partnership is believed to result in empowerment, integration, collaboration, effectiveness, increased satisfaction, quality enhancements, innovation, learning, improvements, and enhanced services within the partnering institutions. When these results are realized, the positive outcomes form the basis for a sustained partnership. In the event that expected results are not achieved, reevaluation of the partnership will result in the need to reassert the essential attributes of the partnership and may also lead to continued unmet needs. Figure 2-1 provides a model of the partnership formation process.

Exemplars of Partnership

The University of Maryland found itself in need of additional faculty, clinical sites for student experiences, additional resources, and employment opportunities for new graduates to ensure the success of its academic program. At the same time, the University of Maryland Medical Center (UMMC) faced the challenges of an increased inpatient census, sicker patients, increased staff vacancies, and a need to provide opportunities for the continuing education of their nurses (University of Maryland School of Nursing, 2007). The two institutions initiated an exploration of each other's needs, assets, and individual visions. When a shared vision emerged, they began to develop a plan with priorities and starting points. Planning evolved with a commitment of resources, sharing of a nurse researcher, and participation of both institutions in research and grant applications. Outcomes from the partnership have included increased clinical experiences for students, increased faculty, integration of the nursing education program and hospital to provide mobile healthcare services to rural areas, and increased enrollment by staff nurses in continuing education initiatives. Data collection on partnership outcomes has allowed formal evaluation of program results and has led to continued modifications and expansion of the program.

The exemplar of the University of Maryland incorporates the antecedent factors of identified needs at an educational and clinical institution and recognition of the need to initiate partnership evaluation. When the essential attributes of trust, respect, openness, and shared values were present, the partnership was formed.

Figure 2–1   Partnership formation process.

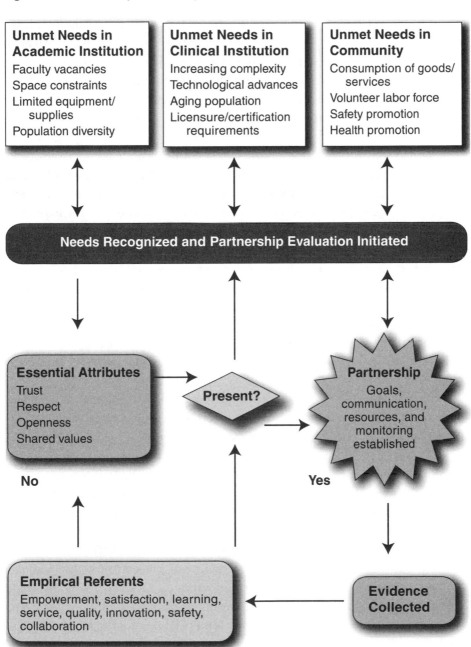

The formation of the partnership progresses with the formation of shared goals, communications, shared resources, and monitoring programs.

In 2004, the Department of Veterans Affairs Medical Centers of the Tennessee Valley Healthcare System (VA TVHS) faced multiple challenges in the provision of patient care. Among these was a fragmented care delivery system that often resulted in frustration for patients, their families, providers, and nurses when patients transitioned from one level of care to another within the system. Nurse managers recognized the need for enhanced multidisciplinary collaboration in the care delivery process, but were often overwhelmed by the operating demands of the units and were unable to focus sufficient attention on clinical care issues. Staff nurses found themselves unable to meet the care needs of their patients because new equipment, advanced information technologies, increased patient acuity, and an aging patient population eroded the amount of time available for individual patients.

Concurrently, Vanderbilt University School of Nursing (VUSN) was facing the challenge presented by rapid technological advances, demands from employing institutions to produce highly skilled and educated nurse generalists who could direct the care of patient populations rather than diagnostic groups. An education focus group was formed including hospitals, educators, and members of the community to identify future nurse management needs. The result of the partnership between VA TVHS and VUSN was the initiation of the CNL role with the first CNLs graduating from VUSN in August 2005.

Community involvement and participation was evident in the implementation of the CNL role as VUSN customized their program to address special needs of the United States Air Force Academy. Additionally, VA TVHS, VUSN, the VA Office of Nursing Services, and AACN collaborated to produce a video for national distribution explaining the CNL role. In 2006, VA TVHS and VUSN began a pilot study for evaluation of empirical referents for successful implementation of the CNL role as developed in collaboration between AACN and the Department of Veterans Affairs. Although the results indicated significant improvement in financial and satisfaction indicators (Hix, McKeon, & Walters, 2009), success of the clinical, academic, and community partnership could be evidenced by joint participation of partners in scholarly publishing activities. Additional activities could include presentations at national conferences, mentorship activities for CNLs from throughout the country, and even the joint celebration of special events and holidays.

Sustaining Partnerships

The lack of progress in changing the delivery of health care to match the complexity of patient needs has been attributed to failure to recognize interdependencies (Wiggins, 2006). Partnerships offer organizations the opportunity to not only recognize interdependencies, but to embrace them as providing mechanisms for effecting positive changes. Examination of the elements of successful partnerships in the implementation of the CNL role has provided insights into strategies that offer the potential to sustain these relationships.

Contract negotiations for student placement in clinical settings present an opportunity to incorporate evidence-based practice outcomes such as review or development of practice guidelines. Nurse executives can influence course content through discussion of important clinical and administrative issues (Newhouse, 2007).

An example of the partnership experience of leaders at the Hunterdon Medical Center and the College of New Jersey at Ewing led to recommendations for sustaining the partnership through frequent open dialogue, openness to learning, and close collaboration. Specific recommendations included that meetings be held on a monthly or other regular schedule; include the chief nursing officer, faculty, and other academic administrators; and that students and other practice stakeholders meet and provide feedback regarding education or implementation matters (Rusch & Bakewell-Sachs, 2007).

> "I have found no greater satisfaction than achieving success through honest dealing and strict adherence to the view that, for you to gain, those you deal with should gain as well."
>
> Alan Greenspan

The extent to which academic, clinical, and community partnerships are able to be maintained depends in part on the investment in efforts to understand the culture and values of the individual organizational participants. To this end, feedback between and among all stakeholders must be sought and given with the goal of continuously improving outcomes. Although activities such as curriculum development, orientation of students and faculty, and assessment and improvement of performance are critical to evaluation and implementation, it is equally important to maintain a focus on the relationships within the partnership. In this manner, celebrating success, recognizing achievements, and sharing the credit for what is accomplished are essential to the establishment of a common culture and keeping the spirit of the partnership alive.

Summary

- The formation of partnerships begins with recognition of unmet needs and challenges within and between the academic, clinical, and community entities.
- The collection of data and stakeholder input form the basis for a gap analysis that can be used to initiate dialogue for negotiation of the partnership.
- Only when trust, respect, shared values, and openness are present will the partnership be able to move forward.
- In the implementation phase, partnership goals, communication strategies, resources, and monitoring mechanisms are determined.
- As the work of the partnership progresses, evidence is collected for use in outcome evaluation.
- Empirical referents as indicators of the results of the partnership are then evaluated, analyzed, and shared among partners and stakeholders.
- If essential attributes of the partnership continue to be in place, the process of goal revision and review of needs is undertaken as the partnership is sustained.
- As the partnership continues, activities such as publishing results of the work, joining to provide recognition to staff, and celebrating success are important to maintaining the relationship between organizations.

Reflection Questions

1. Focus has been maintained on the establishing and maintaining partnerships between and among nursing organizations and the community. What, if any, changes would you expect in the partnership model if the partnerships were interprofessional, as might occur between a medical school and a hospital?
2. Formal relationships between institutions are not always possible or necessary. What types of collaborative initiatives could a CNL engage in with other healthcare institutions in the community? What types of indicators could be used as empirical referents?

Learning Activities

1. Conduct a needs assessment of a microsystem in a healthcare facility. Use the gap analysis outline to guide your work.
2. Working with your CNL preceptor, identify with your preceptor how each partner benefits from the academic-clinical relationship.

References

American Association of Colleges of Nursing (AACN). (2007). *Implementing a new nursing role—the clinical nurse leader for improved patient care outcomes: Final report of the CNL implementation task force.* Retrieved February 2, 2009, from http://www.aacn.nche.edu/CNL/pdf/MemReport02-2007.pdf

American heritage college dictionary (4th ed.). (2007). Boston: Houghton Mifflin.

Bartels, J. (2005). Educating nurses for the 21st century. *Nursing and Health Sciences, 7*(4), 221–225.

Bartels, J., & Bednash, G. (2005). Answering the call for quality nursing care and patient safety. *Nursing Administration Quarterly, 29*(1), 5–13.

Cheung, R., & Aiken, L. (2006). Hospital initiatives to support a better-educated workforce. *Journal of Nursing Administration, 36*(7/8), 357–362.

Gallant, M. H., Beaulieu, M. C., & Carnevale, F. A. (2002). Partnership: An analysis of the concept within the nurse-client relationship. *Journal of Advanced Nursing, 40*(2), 149–157.

Hix, C., McKeon, L., & Walters, S. (2009). Clinical nurse leader impact on clinical microsystems outcomes. *Journal of Nursing Administration, 39*(2), 71–76.

Hook, M. L. (2006). Partnering with patients—a concept ready for action. *Journal of Advanced Nursing, 56*(2), 133–143.

Institute of Medicine (IOM). (2000). *To err is human: Building a safer health system.* Washington, DC: National Academies of Science.

Kerfoot, K., Rapala, K., Ebright, P., & Rogers, S. (2006). The power of collaboration with patient safety programs: Building safe passage for patients, nurses and clinical staff. *Journal of Nursing Administration, 36*(12), 582–588.

Kimball, B., & O'Neil, E. (2002). *Health care's human crisis: The American nursing shortage.* Princeton, NJ: Robert Wood Johnson Foundation.

Merriam-Webster online dictionary. (2008). Retrieved February 17, 2009, from http://www.merriam-webster.com

National League for Nursing, Board of Governors. (2003). *Position statement: Innovation in nursing education: A call to reform.* Retrieved February 2, 2009, from http://www.nln.org/aboutnln/PositionStatements/innovation.htm

Newhouse, R. P. (2007). Collaborative synergy: Practice and academic partnerships in evidence-based practice. *Journal of Nursing Administration, 37*(3), 105–108.

Pew Health Professions Commission. (1998). *Recreating health professional practice for a new century: The fourth report of the Pew Health Professions Commission.* San Francisco: Author. Retrieved January 15, 2009, from http://www.futurehealth.ucsf.edu/pdf_files/recreate.pdf

Rusch, L., & Bakewell-Sachs, S. (2007). The CNL: A gateway to better care? *Nursing Management, 48*(4), 32–40.

Stanley, J. M., Hoiting, T., Burton, D., Harris, J., & Norman, L. (2007). Implementing innovation through education-practice partnerships. *Nursing Outlook, 55*(2), 67–73.

Stark, P. (2003). Clinical teaching and learning in the clinical setting: A qualitative study of the perceptions of students and teachers. *Medical Education, 37*(11), 975–982.

Steinhart, C. M., & Alsup, R. G. (2001, May). Partnerships in health care: Creating a strong value chain. *Physician Executive.* Retrieved February 10, 2009, from http://findarticles.com/p/articles/mi_m0843/is_3_27/ai_75451945

University of Maryland School of Nursing, Office of Communications. (2007). *Nursing: Leadership, partnership, innovation* (pp. 1–30). Baltimore: Author. Retrieved February 1, 2009, from http://nursing.umaryland.edu/docs/publications/UM-NURSING-Sprg07.pdf

Vallejo, P., Saura, R. M., Sunol, R., Kazandjian, V., Urena, V., & Mauri, J. (2006). A proposed adaptation of the EFQM fundamental concepts of excellence to health care based on the PATH framework. *International Journal for Quality in Health Care, 18*(5), 327–335.

Wiggins, M. (2006). The partnership care delivery model. *Journal of Nursing Administration, 36*(7/8), 341–345.

Zahner, S., & Gredig, Q. (2005). Improving public health nursing education: Recommendations of local public health nurses. *Public Health Nursing, 22*(5), 445–450.

THREE

Preparing Clinical Preceptors

■ Sandra E. Walters and Stephanie S. Brown

■ Learning Objectives

- ■ Identify CNL roles in preceptorship.
- ■ Identify core values for the CNL in becoming a preceptor.
- ■ Identify core competencies needed for the CNL as a preceptor.
- ■ Define preceptorship.
- ■ Identify a model for use by clinical preceptors.
- ■ Identify an exemplar of preceptorships in the implementation of the CNL role.

"As the true object of education is not to render the pupil a mere copy of his preceptor, it is rather to be rejoiced in, than lamented, that various readings should lead him into new trains of thinking . . . "

William Godwin

Key Terms

Preceptor	Pupil
Instructor	Mentee
Mentor	Apprentice

CNL Roles

Educator
Member of a profession

CNL Professional Values

Altruism	Human dignity
Integrity	

CNL Core Competencies

Communication	Critical thinking

Introduction

In 2002, the Joint Commission on Accreditation of Healthcare Organizations (JCAHO), now called The Joint Commission, issued recommendations for aligning nursing education and clinical experience as a means for addressing the nursing shortage. In 2007, in its *White Paper on the Role and Education of the Clinical Nurse Leader*, the American Association of Colleges of Nursing (AACN) recognized that a simple increase in the number of nurses would not suffice, and that instead the nursing profession must produce graduates who contribute to the profession by practicing at the full scope of their education and ability. Among the roles of the CNL identified by AACN, that of *educator* makes the CNL responsible for supervising and evaluating other healthcare personnel. This makes it essential for the CNL to develop and maintain skills as a clinical preceptor. Additionally, the role of the CNL as a *member of a profession* makes the CNL accountable for acquisition of skills and knowledge to effect changes in the profession. Functioning as a preceptor provides the CNL with a mechanism to ensure evidence-based practice at the point of care and thus make a positive impact on the profession of nursing.

The transition of nurses from education to practice settings has long been recognized as producing high levels of stress for new graduates. As the CNL enters the healthcare system, it is expected that the new role will provide a mechanism to support nursing education initiatives aimed at making the role transition for novice nurses easier.

Among the values to which CNLs must be committed, those of altruism, human dignity and integrity are critical to the ability of the CNL to function effectively in the role of a preceptor. *Altruism*, the concern for the welfare of others allows the CNL to develop an understanding of the cultures, beliefs, and perspectives of other persons. The willingness to take risks on behalf of clients and colleagues will provide a strong foundation for protective actions undertaken as a preceptor.

Human dignity is the value that allows the CNL to view each individual as unique and to ascribe to each inherent worth. Actions of the CNL as a preceptor will be supported by the CNL's efforts to protect the privacy and confidentiality of others and to design interventions that reflect compassion and sensitivity.

Integrity, maintaining accepted standards of practice and ethical conduct, are essential to the preceptor role because the CNL must provide honest and accurate appraisal of the care delivered by others. By demonstrated accountability through actions such as identifying and correcting errors, documenting accurately, and providing honest information, the CNL will be able to gain the trust and respect of the individuals they are a preceptor to, and this will enhance their effectiveness.

Concurrently, the CNL will be expected to lead experienced nurses to better function as preceptors to less experienced staff (AACN, 2007). In order for this goal to be realized, the role of the CNL will require assimilation of the preceptor role.

> "As the man who digs obtains water by use of a shovel, so the student attains the knowledge possessed by his preceptor through his service."
>
> Chanakya Pandit

Defining Preceptorship

The *American Heritage Dictionary* (2007) defines *preceptorship* as "a period of practical experience and training for a student, especially of medicine or nursing that is supervised by an expert or specialist in a particular field." The related terms *preceptor* and *precept* were adopted in the 14th century from the Latin words *praeceptum* and *praecipere,* which meant to admonish or teach (*Merriam-Webster Online Dictionary*, 2008).

Many individuals use the terms *teacher*, *mentor*, and *preceptor* synonymously, but a distinction should be made to clarify these. A teacher is someone who instructs or imparts knowledge to an individual or a group, with knowledge going predominantly from the teacher to the student or pupil. There is no personal relationship implied except as an instructor/learner dyad, and the teacher and students are often assigned. Whereas a mentor also imparts knowledge, this implies a relationship between two individuals in which both often agree to be actors. The less formal mentor/mentee relationship often spans the length of a career or lifetime, and both the mentor and mentee help determine the course of information and evaluation. Like the mentor relationship, the preceptor/preceptee (or protégé) relationship is also between two individuals but is more formal. The individuals are often assigned, have specific goals, and are generally together for a shorter duration (as in a year or semester). The core competencies of the CNL, as identified by AACN, must all be integrated into the abilities of preceptors because they define the essential components of the CNL's skills and abilities. Nonetheless, the preceptor function requires that the critical thinking and communication abilities of the CNL be applied at a higher level of complexity.

Critical thinking is essential to the preceptor role because the CNL applies research, theories, and models to nursing practice. In using critical thinking, the CNL must be able to evaluate practice and make decisions while considering multiple perspectives regarding issues and problems identified. This skill will facilitate reflection on the outcomes of care given and will allow meaningful dialogue with others regarding professional practice. In effect, one of the primary goals of a preceptor is to assist in the development of critical thinking skills in others and is thus an essential element in the preceptor's competencies.

Communication is a complex process that will allow the CNL to impart and receive information through a variety of mechanisms. As a preceptor, the CNL must be able to interpret oral, written, and nonverbal communications. Communications themselves may require a high level of technological skills because modalities include videoconferencing, computerized applications, and a wide array of personal devices. Additionally, the ability to express ideas in a clear, effective manner to maintain positive relationships is critical to the preceptor function. The CNL focus is believed to be primarily that of a preceptor/preceptee in this writing.

Box 3-1   EBP Toolbox

Specific indicators for performance should provide clearly defined expectations that are objective and measurable. The following can be used to classify performance levels.

1. *Identified limitation*: requires direct guidance with skill
2. *Capable*: familiar but needs some support with unfamiliar skill
3. *Performs independently*: performs safely; often goal of preceptorship
4. *Proficient*: extensive experience and can teach others
5. *Expert*: develops thinking in others + assures evidence-based practice

Model for Clinical Preceptors

Although studies demonstrate that retention of nurses can be improved through the use of preceptor programs, there has been less of a focus on specific strategies to be used. A meta-analysis conducted by Salt, Cummings, and Profetto-McGrath (2008) compared preceptor models and demonstrated that retention strategies that focused on the new graduate nurse showed higher retention rates than those that focused on the experience of the clinical preceptors. Regardless of the focus of the retention strategies, preparation of the preceptor is essential because many expert clinicians lack the ability to function as preceptors.

The focus on the need to increase safety in the healthcare environment has rendered the role of the preceptor as a protector to be essential. Boyer (2008) delineated preceptor responsibilities as including the need to provide a safe learning environment, collect evidence of competence to practice, and build networks for support, communication, and nurturing to take place. The performance and self-assessment key presented by Boyer uses a novice to expert orientation and provides a guide by which to evaluate practice.

The One-Minute Preceptor is a model designed to guide the actions of preceptors in the clinical setting and was originally designed to educate medical residents in family practice. This five-step tool has been used to enhance the skills of nurses in the preceptor role (Kertis, 2007). The steps are presented with an explanation, example, and important aspects for implementation.

The One-Minute Preceptor

Step 1: Get a commitment.

- Have orientee present his/her plan of care or interventions plan for problem.
- Ask: What do you think should be done first?
- It is important to accept orienteer's response without being judgmental.

Step 2: Probe for supporting evidence.

- Establish the knowledge basis for decisions in step 1.
- Ask: What do you think should be done first?
- Ask: Why were these choices made?
- Thinking out loud allows assessment of knowledge and critical thinking skills.

Step 3: Teach general rules.

- Provide correct information or provide location of resources.
- Tell: Provide location of resources and expectations for knowledge or review.
- This step may be omitted if orientee presented all information correctly.

Step 4: Reinforce what was right.

- Provide positive feedback to promote confidence and self-esteem.
- Tell: Specific information regarding what was done.
- Positive praise encourages repeated behavior and imitation by others.

Step 5: Correct mistakes.

- Provide specific information regarding necessary improvement.
- Tell: Improvement needed and rationale.
- It is essential to provide privacy and protect the dignity of the orientee.

Exemplar of Preceptorship

When the first nurses from the VA Tennessee Valley Healthcare System (TVHS) enrolled in the Clinical Nurse Leader (CNL) Program at Vanderbilt University, there were no individuals in the CNL role to serve as preceptors. Master's-prepared nurses who had previously been in the role of case managers transitioned to the role of the CNL. The nurse executive became the preceptor for the CNLs, and soon there were CNLs in multiple settings including ambulatory care, medical/surgical, hospice, rehabilitation, and mental health units. Interest in the CNL role at the national level grew rapidly, and it was a short period of time before other facilities were requesting to visit TVHS to learn about the CNL role.

As the CNLs served as preceptors for CNLs from the region, as well as from distant parts of the country, several lessons were learned regarding the preceptor role. The lessons were extracted from journals maintained by the CNLs and are summarized as follows:

- When staff has been deemed ready to perform independently, it is important to assist them to build confidence in their ability if they disagree.
- Providing a written evaluation plan at the beginning of the preceptorship is critical to maintaining a focus on the level of progress to be attained.
- It is critical that the preceptor act as gatekeeper to prevent the novice from taking on too much responsibility. Sharing expectations with everyone is important as a mechanism by which to limit what others will attempt to assign the novice.
- Celebration of every success is important in serving as publicity, as well as in garnering the interest and support of stakeholders.
- Keeping a journal of the preceptorship experience facilitates program evaluation and encourages self-appraisal for all participants in the preceptorship. It is more important that entries be meaningful than that they be lengthy.

The College of Nursing at University of South Alabama introduced the CNL role and has made it a central focus of its participation in Transforming Care at the Bedside (TCAB), a joint initiative between the Robert Wood Johnson Foundation, the Institute for Healthcare Improvement and the American Organization of Nurse Executives (http://www.ihi.org/IHI/Programs/StrategicInitiatives/TransformingCareAtThe Bedside.htm). The experience in the development of the CNL preceptor in the clinical partner institution resulted in the identification of additional skill sets necessary for preceptors including:

- Willingness to let go of initiatives that were previously tightly controlled;
- Understanding that although the CNL may focus on the microsystem, an understanding of the macrosytem is essential as well;
- Ability to be a champion in preceptorship without the need to take over;
- A willingness to learn while engaged as a preceptor;
- Ability to assist others to reach out to those around them; and
- A sense of humor.

"A disciple attains prominence by carrying out the orders of his preceptors, given with the intention of illuminating his intellect—however harsh they might be. Even though a gem found in a mine might be precious, it needs to undergo the rigors of a grindstone, before it adorns the crown of monarchs."

English Translation of Sanskrit Quote

Summary

- For the CNL, the ability to incorporate the roles of educator and member of a profession into the preceptor experience will require the application of the values of altruism, human dignity, and integrity.
- Both communication and critical thinking skills are identified as essential for successful preceptorships and can be evaluated using tools such as the Boyer's Evaluation of Practice Criteria.
- The One-Minute Manager provides a succinct manner in which to organize the clinical experiences of staff while offering an uncomplicated approach to the communication process.
- Exemplars of preceptorships have been reviewed with elements of success identified.

Reflection Questions

1. Discuss the difference between the relationships of course faculty and clinical preceptors.
2. Compare the formation of a preceptorship with the development of a partnership as discussed in Chapter 1.

Learning Activities

1. Utilize the One-Minute Preceptor model to "precept" a staff member in a new procedure or one used infrequently. Evaluate strengths and weaknesses in the approach.
2. Working with your preceptor, describe your microsystem's readiness for change. Identify tools to assist with recognition of strengths and barriers to success in your CNL-precepted experience.

References

American Association of Colleges of Nursing (AACN). (2007). *White paper on the education and role of the clinical nurse leader*. Retrieved February 10, 2009, from http://www.aacn.nche. edu/Publications/WhitePapers/ClinicalNurseLeader.htm

American heritage college dictionary (4th ed.). (2007). Boston: Houghton Mifflin.

Boyer, S. A. (2008). Competence and innovation in preceptor development: Updating our programs. *Journal for Nurses in Staff Development, 24*(2), E1–E6.

The Joint Commission. (2002). *Health care at the crossroads: Strategies for addressing the evolving nursing crisis*. Chicago: Author.

Kertis, M. (2007). The One-Minute Preceptor: A five-step tool to improve clinical teaching skills. *Journal for Nurses in Staff Development, 23*(5), 238–242.

Merriam-Webster online dictionary. (2008). Retrieved February 17, 2009, from http://www.-merriam-webster.com

Salt, J., Cummings, G., & Profetto-McGrath, J. (2008). Increasing retention of new graduate nurses: A systematic review of interventions by healthcare organizations. *Journal of Nursing Administration, 38*(6), 297–301.

FOUR

The CNL Advisory Council

■ Karen M. Ott

■ Learning Objectives

- ■ Define the power/relevance of partnership and collaboration to CNL sustainment.
- ■ Describe the role of the CNL Advisory Council.
- ■ Develop a CNL Advisory Council Charter to include outcomes and deliverables.

> "Anyone who proposes to do good must not expect people to roll stones out of his way, but must accept his lot calmly if they even roll a few more upon it."
>
> **Albert Schweitzer**

> "You need to surround yourself with quality human beings that are intelligent and have a vision."
>
> **Vince McMahon**

Key Terms

Advisory councils   Charters
CNL role sustainment

CNL Roles

Consultant   Professional leader

CNL Professional Values

Integrity   critical thinking
Member of a profession

CNL Core Competencies

Communication   Accountability
Interpersonal effectiveness

Introduction

The decision to create a CNL advisory council by an organization may be the single most important decision to ensure sustainment of their CNL program. Much has been written about the challenges an organization faces when a major change is introduced. Introducing a change to the nursing profession presents no less a challenge when the variety of roles are often extensive, duplicative, and overlapping.

The CNL Advisory Council: An Opportunity for Partnership and Collaboration

A CNL advisory council provides a forum for academic and healthcare organizations to engage in synergistic partnership and collaboration. The council's combined knowledge, experience, and vision positions the organization to achieve the best course of action for the integration and sustainment of the CNL program for the long term.

Advisory councils may be established for distinctly different purposes: for example, to provide advice and direction for a specific program or to actively lead the development and formation of policies and processes. This chapter will provide information and guidance for the establishment of advisory councils that serve either purpose. Examples presented throughout the chapter describe aspects of the CNL advisory council that was established by the Office of Nursing Services at the Department of Veterans Affairs. This CNL advisory council was established to lead the formation and implementation of policies and processes intended to advance and sustain the CNL program within the Veterans Health Administration.

Advisory Council Responsibilities

An advisory council's leader, facilitator, and members each have distinct roles. The following sections identify the key responsibilities of each role.

The Leader

The leader drives the council's organization and development and serves as its primary point of contact with the organization's formal leadership. Additionally, the leader's responsibilities include the following:

- Overseeing the development and implementation of the council charter including the goals (may be shared with a facilitator);
- Recruiting and orienting members;
- Planning meetings (monthly or quarterly);
- Overseeing council operations;
- Ensuring effective council structure, roles and processes; and
- Evaluating the effectiveness of the council.

The Facilitator

According to Ball & Associates, an advisory council is best served when there is an environment of collaborative tension (Ball & Associates, n.d.). A facilitator can balance the effectiveness of interactions (process) and initiatives/action items (content) to achieve a synergistic partnership. The leader would consider the following when making the decision about whether to use a facilitator (see Table 4-1).

Table 4-1   Considerations for the Use of a Facilitator

A Facilitator Is Needed	A Facilitator Is Not Needed
Council members are not a previously formed group, accountable to each other, nor will likely work interdependently on a regular basis.	Council members are a formed and cohesive team.
The purpose and the goals are not clearly understood.	Members share a solid and recognized commitment to the purpose and goals.
Neither group process nor content is clearly understood.	Members understand group methods, tools, and the topics under discussion.
The leader does not possess facilitation skills.	The leader is skilled in negotiating, evoking response, and recognizing group dynamics.
The leader wants to maximize the group's participation in all aspects of the meeting	The leader is able to fully participate, observe, and orchestrate process and content to meet desired outcomes.
There are complex issues with multiple possible solutions and potential for conflict.	The leader can remain objective and has no vested interest in one course of action over another.

Source: Adapted from Ball & Associates, 2009.

The Members

Advisory councils typically do not function independently nor have legal authority; therefore, the initiatives and action items of the members may require leadership approval before implementation (McNamara, n.d.).

Members' responsibilities include the following.

- *Program Planning and Review.* A small group of members may be valuable advisors in the early stages of CNL program planning and design. Council membership can be expanded at a later time.
- *Policy and Protocol Creation.* Members agree to take responsibility for the development of policies and protocols that will provide direction and support for the CNL program goals.

- *Subcommittees.* Members agree to establish and lead subcommittees to accomplish assigned tasks in specific areas, in specified timeframes.
- *Marketing and Communication.* Members can be effective and influential champions for the CNL role both within and outside of the organization.

Subcommittees

It is advisable to establish subcommittees to assist with the development of council goals, especially goals that are complex or long term. Subcommittees should be led by a council member with additional council members participating, as needed. Each subcommittee must have a specific charge or set of tasks to address. All subcommittee recommendations for policy and process should be approved by the entire council. Whether established as continuing (for the duration of the goal) or ad hoc (one-time), subcommittees can provide valuable expertise and diversity for the council (NcNamara, n.d.).

Getting Started

The leader's primary responsibilities include the following:

Draft the Charter

A charter serves two main objectives: to formally establish a council and clarify its purpose, and to identify its goals. A typical charter contains seven headings: Purpose; Charge (goals); Chair; Membership; Terms (duration); Reporting Requirements (interaction with the organizational leadership); and Meetings (types/frequency).

Recruit Members

As previously stated, the strength and effectiveness of an advisory council lies in the commitment, contribution, and influence of its members. Leaders must recruit and select members that "can engage with the topic, build understanding, create new ideas, support each other, bring the outside world into the group, and the work of the group to the outside world" (Ball & Associates, n.d.).

The following recruiting guidelines from Carter McNamara can make the recruitment process more effective (McNamara, n.d). The leader should consider the following actions:

- *Develop and distribute a questionnaire or application form that will serve to recruit prospective council members.* In addition to asking for basic biographical information, include questions that will solicit their purpose in

Table 4-2   Sample CNL Advisory Council Charter

Purpose: Develop and implement initiatives to fully integrate and sustain the CNL role in all patient care settings in every VA medical center by 2016.

Charge: *May include outcomes and deliverables*

- Develop a CNL residency/fellowship program to augment the postgraduate orientation and mentoring of newly graduated CNLs.
- Develop a national patient-driven nursing care delivery model centered on the CNL role.
- Initiate a salary replacement program for CNL master's completion.
- Fully implement the CNL role at the five VA regional polytrauma medical centers.
- Develop national CNL performance measures.
- Enable CNL outcomes to be readily identifiable in the VA Nursing Outcomes Database (VANA).
- Develop a CNL/Advanced Practice RN (APRN) business plan template.
- Revise the CNL position description and core competencies template.

Membership: (Practice and Academic Partners)

Chair: May have co-chairs from practice and academic partners

Meeting Requirements: *Types/frequency*

Initial meeting scheduled as a face-to-face. Subsequent meetings via conference calls and face-to-face as needed. Work will be predominately conducted by members outside scheduled conference calls.

Reporting Requirements: *Reporting schedule details*

Updates provided to the chief nursing officer 2 weeks following the initial meetings and monthly afterward until project completion.

---

applying for membership, their relevant personal and professional goals, and their value to the council and to its goals. Identify the terms and conditions of membership—for example, term length, role, and responsibilities.

- *Keep an updated list of prospective council members.* Solicit information about members' position, scope of responsibility, and the skills they possess relevant to both the organization's strategic goals and the council's goals.
- *Meet with prospective council members.* Interview the nominees who are being considered for selection to acquaint them with the role and responsibilities of the members and to identify any conflicts of interest or potential negative issues.

- *Invite prospective members to council meetings.* Help the prospective member become acquainted with other council members and with council business.
- *Contact prospective members afterward.* Determine whether the member is still interested in becoming an advisory council member, and provide appropriate follow-up action with organizational leadership if higher concurrence is required.
- *Provide new member orientation.* Notify council members of actions taken.

Plan and Organize the Meeting

A well-planned and organized meeting requires the leader (with the facilitator, if applicable) to set meeting goals, identify participants, attend to logistical support, and draft and distribute the agenda (Burke et al., 2002). When planning the meeting, the leader should consider the following:

- *Goals.*
  What are the overarching goals for the meeting?
  What specifically needs to be accomplished at the meeting?
  How much time is needed for each goal or task to be accomplished?
- *Participants.*
  Are the right people invited?
  Can everyone participate as needed?
- *Logistical support.*
  What meeting space and A/V equipment need to be obtained?
  Does the agenda require a working lunch?
  Does lodging need to be identified/reserved?
  Do maps/directions need to be developed and distributed?
- *The meeting agenda.*
  The agenda should cover the following:
  - Identify the goals, date, time, location, and list of tasks to be accomplished.
  - Be distributed 1 to 2 weeks before the meeting to allow members to understand the expectations and prepare for what's ahead.
  - Allocate a block of time for each group of tasks, or allocate a specific time for each task:
    - Using block time-setting creates a stimulating environment for idea development, especially at the initial meeting.
    - Allocating specific time-setting assures that meeting goals will be met and is best used for subsequent meetings.

Table 4-3   Sample CNL Advisory Council Meeting Agenda:
The Veterans Health Administration

CNL Advisory Council Meeting
Initial Meeting
Date

Meeting Objectives:
- Clarify charter goals/membership
- Identify additional goals
- Prioritize goals
- Identify required action
- Set timelines
- Establish subgroups
- Begin subgroup work
- Identify follow-up requirements

Tuesday, 9/30	Task	Location
8–11:30	1. Clarify CNL advisory charter goals and members. 2. Identify/add goals to advisory group as needed. 3. Establish priority for goal accomplishment. 4. Brainstorm initial list of actions needed to meet goals. 5. Identify initial timeline for goal completion.	Room X
11:30–12:30	Lunch	
12:30–4:30	6. Complete list of actions needed to meet goals. 7. Identify subgroups, with additional members if needed, to align with goals. 8. Finalize timeline for goal completion. 9. Initiate subgroup work.	Room X

Wednesday, 10/1	Task	Location
8–11:30	1. Continue subgroup work.	Room X
11:30–Noon	2. Agree on future meeting mode/schedule for continuation of work and follow-up. 3. Adjourn.	

Conduct the Meeting

At a minimum, the leader (or facilitator) should do the following at every meeting (Burke et al., 2002):

- Review the charter, goals, and timelines.
- Identify members' expectations and desires. At the initial meeting, the leader may ask, "When you attend meetings, what lights your fire and what burns you up?"
- Identify members' challenges and successes at every meeting. Ask, "What do you need to get to the next step/complete this task?"
- Refocus the group when situations impede program, such as the following:
  - Persistent sidebar conversations
  - Never-ending discussion
  - Continual delay in returning from breaks
  - Negative conflict
  - Group isn't staying on task.
- Not intervene to refocus the group if all the participants are engaged in productive discussion to redefine goals, initiatives, or timelines, particularly when sufficient and valid information is present.

Evaluate the Meeting

The leader (and facilitator) should objectively evaluate the meeting as close to the conclusion as possible. The following sample meeting evaluation may be used as a guide (Burke et al., 2002):

Table 4-4   Sample Meeting Evaluation Form

Sample Meeting Evaluation

Name (optional):

Date: /   /

Please evaluate the clarity and relevance of the following elements:

Meeting objectives:

_____ Excellent

_____ Above Average

_____ Average

_____ Poor

Comments:

Meeting tasks:

_____ Excellent

_____ Above Average

_____ Average

_____ Poor

Comments:

Time dedicated to each task:

_____ Excellent

_____ Above Average

_____ Average

_____ Poor

Comments:

Please evaluate the knowledge and skill of the facilitator:

_____ Excellent

_____ Above Average

_____ Average

_____ Poor

_____ Not applicable

Comments:

Source: Adapted from Burke et al., 2002.

Follow Through

Leaders should communicate periodically with council members to clarify tasks, identify obstacles, and provide support for the completion of all action items.

Evaluate the Effectiveness of the Council

It is suggested that the leader (with the facilitator) perform an annual self-assessment of the council to determine whether or not the goals and objectives of the council are being met (Campaign Consultation, Inc., n.d.).

Table 4-5   An Advisory Council Self-Assessment Sample

Activity	Strongly Agree	Agree	Disagree	Strongly Disagree	Actions Needed for Improvement
Council Charter Content is clearly stated, easily understood, and up-to-date. Goals are appropriate and relevant. Council responsibilities are clearly stated.					
Council Operations The frequency and length of council meetings are appropriate. The council operates under a clear set of bylaws or rules. Meeting agendas are effectively designed and distributed in advance.					
Leader Responsibilities Membership includes a diversity of skills and experience to meet council goals. Members are kept apprised of direction, support, and approval from the organization's formal leadership. Member conduct reflects leadership effectiveness (attendance, participation, etc.). Members are recognized for their contributions in an appropriate manner. The membership recruitment process is active and ongoing.					
Membership Roles and Responsibilities Members clearly understand their roles and responsibilities. Members understand the goals and direction of the organization. All members have copies of essential documentation including: the original charter and continuous updates, their roles and responsibilities, and terms as members.					
Member Performance Members work together as a team to accomplish council goals. Members treat each other with respect and communicate effectively. Members have established effective subcommittees to achieve specific tasks. Members provide updates and are self-directed to complete the work.					
Subcommittee Roles and Responsibilities The right number and type of subcommittees have been created to accomplish council goals. Each council member is active on at least one subcommittee.					

Source: Adapted from Campaign Consultation, Inc., 2009.

Tools of the Trade: Case Studies

The Veterans' Health Administration

CNL Advisory Council

The Veterans Health Administration CNL Advisory Council was established to continue expansion and support for the national CNL initiative begun in early 2004. The CNL Advisory Council is a 12-member council composed of nurses from multiple VA medical centers and several academic partners assisting on specific initiatives. The following plan of action describes the goals, action, responsible person, status, and timeline dates for project completion:

Table 4-6   The Veterans Health Administration CNL Advisory Council Plan of Action

Goal	Initiative/ Action	Leader(s)	Members	Status	Projected Date of Completion
1. Develop a pre-CNL program for the workplace, with assistance from academic partners, to reduce CNL graduate requirements.	a. Identify pre-CNL tracks (identify nonaffiliated and level 2–4 facilities as pilot sites).	Paula Enna	Maude Marthe Brenda Rachel Dan Kathy Karen Sharon	a. October X Emailed the nurse executives for feedback on barriers and for existing practices. Received a small number of responses; resend.	October X February X December X
	b. Identify academic institutions and reps to assist with curriculum requirements.			Reps at each school are being contacted to determine their interest and the type of CNL program they offer.	March X
				• Identify the ADN/BSN/MSN tracks.	April X
				• Send Pre-CNL fact sheets to the group.	

Goal	Initiative/ Action	Leader(s)	Members	Status	Projected Date of Completion
2. Develop a CNL residency and fellowship program to augment the postgraduate and mentoring of newly graduated CNLs.	a. Establish CNL student preceptorship/coach policy.	Marthe			February X
	b. Develop a CNL orientation, residency, and fellowship program.	Marthe	Sharon	b. Identify practice sites that have implemented the AACN/UHC Residency Program.	May X
				• Make a final decision on academic/ practice site selection for the VA.	January X
				• Reviewing established programs for preceptors. Review for applicability.	February X
				• Establish a subgroup to assist with the development of this initiative. Reviewing the content of existing orientation and residency programs and send out to group.	February X
	c. Develop a CNL mentorship program.			c. Drafting the beginning components of a CNL mentoring document.	March X
2. Integrate the CNL role at the five polytrauma rehabilitation centers.	a. Institute performance measures, outcomes, and specific functions.	Kathy K. (Sharon will assist Shawna)	Paula Kathy C. Enna Pat J. Brenda Dan	a. Shawna has agreed to assist Kathy with the lead for this initiative. She will also identify additional members.	October X

Goal	Initiative/ Action	Leader(s)	Members	Status	Projected Date of Completion
3. Provide guidance to develop VA Nursing Outcomes Database (VANOD) identifiers for CNL outcomes.	a. Solicit CNL input/ideas at the CNL summit.	Karen	Rachel Sharon Sue Marthe	a. Plan module w/Bonnie prior to CNL summit.	January X
				• Bonnie will facilitate a breakout session at the 1/29 CNL summit to obtain feedback that will help her capture CNL outcomes for VANOD.	January X
				• Identify partnership opportunities for CNL outcomes with CNL and physicians.	March X
4. Consultant to the National Nursing Executive Council (NNEC) Nursing Practice Transformation Goal Group will develop a patient-driven nursing care delivery model centered on the CNL role.	a. Propose CNL organizational/ reporting structures.	Marthe Paula	Kathy C. Pat Paula Marthe Dan Enna Maude Sharon	a. Drafting a sample organizational reporting structures for CNLs.	December X
	b. Crosswalk CNL w/CNS, NM, CM, CC, charge nurse, and clinical educator.			b. Preparing to send out the crosswalk info to the group soon.	January X
	c. Review/revise the CNL functional statement and core competencies.			c. Nearly completed with the revised FS and will send out to group.	February X
	d. Identify additional specialty care settings where CNL may achieve very specific outcomes.			d. Developing the role for VA CNLs in additional care settings: gerontology and hospice/palliative care.	August X

Goal	Initiative/ Action	Leader(s)	Members	Status	Projected Date of Completion
	e. Research models of care delivery and CNL impact including appropriate "panel size" of patients/CNL.			e. Soliciting models for care delivery and CNL impact.	January X
				• Plan to examine existing literature regarding CNS, intensivist, and hospitalist models.	February X
5. Create a national deployment/ succession plan for CNL.	a. Identify appropriate performance measures impacted by CNL.	Karen Kathy C.	Enna		October X
	b. Work with VISN for salary replacement dollars with HRRO.			b. Developing a CNL/APRN business plan. First meeting scheduled for 3/10.	March X
6. Build and sustain partnership with major stakeholders.	a. Interdisciplinary team (IDT)	Dan	Paula Karen Sharon Marthe		October X
	b AACN and other professional organizations				
	c. Academic institutions				
	d. VA clinical specialty advisors				
	e. VA Office of Academic Affiliations				
	f. Regulatory and accrediting bodies				
	g. Labor partners				
	h. Compensation agencies (research ways to recognize CNL)				
	i. Magnet culture				

Goal	Initiative/ Action	Leader(s)	Members	Status	Projected Date of Completion
7. Innovative education/ develop practice initiative to sustain the role.		Marthe			June X
8. Create CNL marketing/ "branding."		Karen			June X
9. Explore feasibility of VA-funded research to study CNL patient outcomes.		Maude	Sue		June X

Summary

- The decision to use an advisory council to enhance and sustain the CNL role is paramount to the success of an organization's CNL program.
- The first critical step is the development of a charter with a clearly defined purpose and the identification of major goals.
- Recruiting a diverse group of qualified, visionary, committed members to create and lead an effective course of action does not have to be complicated.

Reflection Questions

1. What key goals or action steps can be achieved by a CNL advisory council?
2. What types of academic and clinical members are best suited for a CNL advisory council?
3. Are there other types of members that will add a valuable dimension to the council's work?

Learning Activities

1. Participate on an established CNL Advisory Council.
2. As a CNL student, describe your observations during a CNL Advisory Council meeting.
3. What are your assessments of members' communication, the decision-making process, and follow-up plans?

References

Ball, G., & Associates. (n.d.). *Geoff Ball & Associates: Enabling people to work together better.* Retrieved March 23, 2009, from http://www.geoffballfacilitator.com/basics.html

Burke, D. W., Donahoe, M., Hirzel, R., Mather, L., Morganstern, G., Ruete, N., et al. (2002). *Basic facilitation skills.* Retrieved March 23, 2009, from http://www.scribd.com/doc/39340/Basic-Facilitation-Skills

Campaign Consultation, Inc. (n.d.). *Advisory council member self-assessment.* Retrieved March 23, 2009, from http://www.nationalserviceresources.org/files/legacy/filemanager/download/forms/VIG1.pdf

McNamara, C. (n.d.). *Facilitation (face-to-face and online).* Retrieved March 23, 2009, from http://managementhelp.org/grp_skll/facltate/facltate.htm

Schuman, S. (moderator). (n.d.). *Facilitator competencies* (from the electronic discussion on group facilitation). Retrieved March 23, 2009, from http://www.albany.edu/cpr/gf/resources/FacilitatorCompetencies.html

White, N. (2004, April 3). *Facilitating and hosting a virtual community.* Retrieved March 23, 2009, from http://www.fullcirc.com/community/communityfacilitation.htm

Unit 3

Readying the Academic and Clinical Environments for the Clinical Nurse Leader: Clinical Experience and Transition

FIVE

The Clinical Nurse Leader as a Transformed Leader

■ Sharon Cannon and Carol Boswell

■ **Learning Objectives**

- Compare several different leadership styles related to focus, power, responsibilities, strengths, and weaknesses.
- Explain key aspects of the CNL role related to leadership styles, change theories, complexity, and microsystem analysis.
- Discuss fundamental concepts related to microsystem analysis.
- Describe how the CNL is a transformational leader.

> "Do not go where the path may lead, go instead where there is no path and leave a trail."
>
> Ralph Waldo Emerson

Key Terms

Chaos theory

Autocratic leadership

Laissez-faire leadership

Participative leader

Succession planning

Nonlinear model

Learning organization theory

Microsystem analysis

Democratic leadership

Consultative leader

Servant leader

Linear model

Change theory

Complexity theory

Transformational leader

CNL Roles

Outcome manager

Educator

Team manager

Lifelong learner

Client advocate

Systems analysis/risk anticipator

Member of a profession

CNL Professional Values

Altruism

Human dignity

Social justice

Accountability

Integrity

CNL Core Competencies

Critical thinking

Ethics

Global health care

Provider and manager of care

Nursing technology and resource
  management

Communication

Human diversity

Healthcare systems and policy

Designer/manager/coordinator of care

Member of a profession

Introduction

Within leadership and management textbooks, questions are often raised relating to whether a leader is born or made. Additional questions revolve around the idea of the following:

1. What qualities must be learned to be a good CNL?
2. Are leadership and management the same thing?
3. If leaders are born, then what is necessary to improve or overcome traits that are characteristics for leading?

When answering these questions, a definition of leadership is needed. According to Barnhart and Stein (1962), a leader is a person who guides and directs movement within a situation. Jooste (2004) stated, "Effective leadership is about enabling ordinary people to produce extraordinary things in the face of challenge and change and to constantly turn in superior performance to the long-term benefit of all concerned" (p. 217). Leadership can be understood to be an individual who has the rank, purpose, or direction that results from the capacity to oversee a state of affairs. Thus, leadership requires an individual who is able to use tasks, skills, and abilities to execute a plan forward toward successful completion.

The American Association of Colleges of Nursing (AACN; 2007) proposed the clinical nurse leader (CNL) role as a response to the changing healthcare delivery environment. The AACN envisioned this role as a clinical leader function that transcends all healthcare settings. According to AACN (2007), "The CNL functions within a micro-system and assumes accountability for healthcare outcomes for a specific group of clients within a unit or setting through the assimilation and application of research-based information to design, implement, and evaluate client plans of care" (p. 6). The CNL is viewed as a contributor to the management of holistic care at the point of care (POC) to individuals and/or clusters of individuals with like healthcare needs. According to Hartranft, Garcia, and Adams (2007), "Providing direct care and clinical leadership at the bedside allows the CNL the opportunity to facilitate patient information, coordinate care between disciplines, identify changes in patient conditions by reviewing laboratory results and radiology reports through patient rounds, and provide education to staff, patients, and families" (p. 262). The AACN describes ten assumptions for the preparation of the CNL. For example, the CNL's practice is at the microsystems level, focusing on client care outcomes based on evidence used to measure quality practice. Good fiscal stewardship is essential to quality care, with social justice as an essential nursing value. The CNL's practice is client-centered and is intra- and interdisciplinary. The CNL uses information to maximize self-care and client decision making focusing on nursing assessment as the basis for theory and knowledge development. Lastly, communication technology for the CNL facilitates continuity and comprehensiveness of care. First and foremost, the CNL assumes guardianship for the nursing profession. As these assumptions are implemented into a serviceable designation, certain aspects of the role must be carefully considered and developed.

Concerns about the nursing shortage and the aging workforce present a challenge for managers to develop staff to assume clinical nursing leadership positions. Development of the CNL is of paramount importance as clinical experts and seasoned leaders navigating the complex healthcare delivery environment leave the workforce. Departure of expert leaders will leave a void if CNLs are not mentored and developed as this critical changeover progresses. Peck (2007) stated that "we need new strategies to help the next generation of leaders deal with the gale-force winds of change in the global marketplace" (p. 1). The clinical leader for the next generation must be able to dominate the turbulence and complexity of the healthcare environment while maintaining the momentum of change within the nursing profession. Successful management of the chaos and complexity confronting health care and the nursing profession can be used as forces for incremental and transformational change. "Transformational leaders who break out of old and relied upon patterns and create different ones will occur as roles are recognized and their impact is validated by appreciable outcomes" (Sheldon Rovin, personal communication, October 5, 2006).

Leadership Styles

According to Longest (2004), "Although research shows that possession of certain traits alone does not guarantee leadership success, there is evidence that effective leaders are different from other people in certain key respects" (p. 132). The key leader traits for incorporation include the following: drive that includes accomplishment, motivation, aspiration, energy, persistence, and initiative; leadership motivation that represents the yearning to guide without the requirement of control and power; honesty and integrity; self-confidence that includes emotional steadiness; cognitive ability; and knowledge. As a clinical leader selects the techniques of leadership he or she feels comfortable with, these key traits should be thoughtfully considered and assessed. A leader can fluctuate from one leadership style to another based on the setting and situation, but each finds a primary leadership style that is the most comfortable.

Traditional Styles

There are many different leadership styles, but three methods of leadership are considered to be traditional systems frequently integral within the workplace: autocratic, democratic, and laissez-faire. CNLs must be knowledgeable of each when assuming roles and partnering with the nurse manager.

Autocratic leadership is seen as a "take charge" type of management. Each step within the management and conduction of business affairs is directed and controlled by the individual assuming the leadership position. The person in charge does not seek input but rather depends on pronouncing which tasks and/or business will be completed. He or she accepts the responsibility for prioritizing all of the activities of the group or agency. The role of others within the organization is to accept the directives provided by the leader and carry them out without any opportunity to interject suggestions, comments, or alter decisions.

A second traditional leadership style for discussion is the democratic method. Within this mode of leadership, opinions, suggestions, and concerns of the employees are sought and considered in the decision-making process. The CNL is pivotal to assimilating staff input and working with the partnering nurse manager to implement change and creative projects at the microsystem level. According to Yoder-Wise and Kowalski (2006), this method "supports independence of the workers and consensus building" (p. 473). The leader values the information provided by colleagues and peers. The leader is required to identify and delineate the boundaries of the situation and/or problem under consideration. Once the limits of the situation are established, each employee is engaged in the determination of a solution for the identified challenge. The group comes up with the solution, rather than having the solution dictated by the leader.

The final traditional leadership style is labeled as laissez-faire. Within this method, the leader is viewed as uninvolved and indecisive. Decisions are pushed down from management to the employee level. The roles within this style are viewed as being indistinguishable. Because no one takes the responsibility for the outcomes, everyone tends to do what they perceive is best. This movement tends to be a protective mechanism because each member of the organization realizes that he or she is without any power yet expected to take responsibility and blame. Laissez-faire is viewed as a "hands-off" type of leadership style.

Nontraditional Styles

Nontraditional styles provide additional ways of considering leadership. Cognizant of leadership styles, the CNL finds the venue that is individually comfortable. Clinical leaders tend to have certain characteristics that reflect a style of leading supportive of the development and growth of others. One such style is the consultative leader. Consultative leaders use explanation and rationales to convince participants to follow decisions. This style provides guidance and understanding, thus allowing decisions grounded on a strong knowledge base.

A second nontraditional style employed by leaders can be participative leadership. Longest (2004) purports that this style allows for the presentation of tentative decisions and/or solutions that facilitate change. The change is allowed when a convincing case is presented reflecting a different decision. This style weighs heavily on participation rather than authority. CNLs are the catalyst for proposing and effecting change based on input from staff and the treatment team.

A final nontraditional style for consideration is the servant leader. A servant leader strives to serve individuals within the group. Characteristics of listening, empathy, healing, awareness, persuasion, conceptualization, foresight, stewardship, commitment, and community building are empowered by the leader. The leader's focus is on group members' needs. As nurses face crises, the ideas within this style of leadership can be thoughtfully considered. Coaching and mentoring of colleagues are integral aspects of the process as CNLs develop and complete meaningful projects.

Key Leadership Issues

When considering leadership styles, succession planning, retention, recruitment, effective characteristics of leaders, and emerging roles are also important to transforming organizations . Beyers (2006) notes, "The turbulence in the environment, the focus on cost and on finances, the need to downsize, to advance technology, and other changes are obstacles to be overcome by leaders who are committed to leadership development" (p. 11). Current strategies to bundle services for reimbursement are an example of how financial aspects and accreditation influence the style of the leader impacting the role and functions of the CNL.

Given the growing crises in nursing clinical leadership, succession planning must be embraced to allow for organizational continuity, securing tactical and operational efficacy. Succession planning is relatively new in nursing leadership; leaders must accept the challenge to educate the parent organization of the value of transitioning to a strong associate carrying the mission and vision of the organization. It should not be left to chance. Thies and Ayers (2007) report, "The working relationship among the two or three frontline players at any point in a delivery system is key to a successful outcome and reflects the shared purpose and information" (p. 326). All need involvement and must work from the same page to ensure continuity of care and advancement of the profession. The CNL is unit-based, and opportunities for coaching and mentoring of staff to assume various roles in their career paths are readily available.

Change Theories

As the CNL identifies the leadership style of the partnering nurse manager, other aspects are considered. The first aspect to be examined is change. Although the term *change* may have some universal meaning for everyone, a clear, common definition of change is important. An acceptable definition for *change* is "to make different" (*Webster's II New College Dictionary*, 1999, p. 186). Different forces are impacting health care today. Thus, clinical leaders must be cognizant of models of change and the roles of the leader associated with the models.

Whether change occurs internally or externally, two models of change determine the approach. The first model is one of planned change. Planned change models are often termed *linear models*. Change, in this model, is thought to take incremental steps in a specific direction, with systematic decisions effecting methods to accomplish the change. Lewin (1947), Lippitt, Watson, and Westley (1958), Havilock (1973), and Rogers (1983) are considered to be classic proponents of planned change models.

Linear Models

Lewin (1947) examined the need for assessing the barriers and facilitators for change. Barriers need to be removed or used to support the facilitators. Lewin's model describes three stages of change: unfreezing, moving, and refreezing.

Resistance to unfreezing comes when individuals do not think change is necessary. A common response during this stage is, "Why do we need to change? We've always done it this way" or "If it's not broke, don't fix it." The effective leader assesses readiness for change and is prepared to motivate individuals to see the need for change.

The moving phase of change notes that change is not enough. The leader has a plan and strategies for implementation. The plan and strategies to put the plan in place are necessary in eliminating barriers and fostering trust in the team. The team needs to perceive the change as one in which they want to participate and assume ownership for the change. Sometimes the leader approaches one or two team members to elicit their support so they can gather support from others. The more members who agree to the change, the more likely the change will occur. Change does not happen overnight. Allowing time for the change and setting timelines is critical. Team members require time, which necessitates that leaders allow for this transition.

Refreezing denotes that once change has been accepted, reinforcement for acceptance of the change is necessary. The idea is to make the change the new status quo (Morgan, Johnson, & Garrison, 2007). At this point, the team becomes comfortable with the change.

In 1958, Lippitt adapted Lewin's theory by putting more emphasis on the role of the change agent. Lippitt included seven steps for the change agent to be successful. Like Lewin, Lippitt proposed that a problem must be recognized so that there is motivation for the changes to occur. The change agent must have the capacity to change, bring about change in others, and be willing to commit money, time, and energy to accomplish the change. Lippitt also believed in incremental steps that require a flexible plan to include evaluation of the process in order for the change to be integrated, maintained, and adapted as needed. In Lippitt's theory, the change agent becomes a team member and not the leader when the change has stabilized.

Havilock's (1973) theory focused primarily on the planning stage through participation by all involved in the change. Again, the more people who believe that the change is necessary, the more likely the change will occur. Similar to Lewin and Lippitt, Havilock suggested that planning requires a relationship of members, identification of the problem, and resources. Movement toward change includes obtaining a solution and gaining acceptance. Finally, the change becomes acceptable.

Rogers (1983) introduced a change theory that includes the concept of diffusion. Rogers paired diffusion with innovation as a process for a new need for a change (innovation) that is communicated to multiple persons throughout a system. Rogers also proposed that the nature of change is reversible. Change may or may not occur, and even if the change is accepted, it may not be maintained. Rogers's theory suggested that when reinforcement does not take place, a decision may be reversed if it cannot be confirmed that the decision was correct.

Nonlinear Models

As cited in Yoder-Wise (2007), "Change is inevitable and unrelenting" (p. 123). Today, in health care, change is happening so fast that linear models may not be the right approach for managing change effectively. Two new major models have emerged and are gaining widespread acceptance by leaders in health care.

The first model to be considered is one involving systems. Another term for systems theory is "learning organization theory." This theory is based on the fact that the whole is more than just the sum of its parts. Each part makes a distinctive contribution to the whole.

Perhaps the best-known learning organization theory is one identified by Peter Senge (1990). This theory allows all members the opportunity to participate while acknowledging that differences within are not only acceptable but encouraged. Senge spoke of five disciplines that must be accomplished. The first discipline is one of personal mastery that requires the members of an organization to develop a vision. Once the vision is developed, the second discipline is for determining a member's belief about the world. Then, those beliefs will result in change, which in turn builds new mental models. The third discipline requires all members to collectively convert their personal vision to a common vision. This discipline takes time for consensus of the group while still recognizing differences may occur. The fourth discipline is for the team to learn and grow together. No one person is the leader, but rather all members participate in decision making. Building a learning team requires putting aside judgments and utilizing effective communication skills, such as active listening, without pointing fingers or placing blame. The fifth, and final, discipline, systems thinking, sometimes becomes the hardest to accomplish. Few would argue that putting theory to practice is a difficult task. Yet, systems thinking is the tie that binds the other four disciplines. The major emphasis of this discipline is to not look at the parts but rather at the whole. Systems thinking acknowledges complexity, infrastructure, patterns, trends, and relationships.

When considering systems theory, one should keep in mind that systems may be closed or open. A closed system is internal or, put another way, self-contained. An open system is one in which forces, both internal and external, apply pressure to generate changes. Sometimes internal changes bring about external changes. Thus, changes can seem to occur from multiple forces and may appear numerous and random. This has resulted in a chaos theory, which suggests unpredictability, with constant change bombarding the organization and its members. Health care can best be described as chaotic. Examples include variables such as an increase in the aging population, Medicare reimbursement issues, accrediting organizations' requirements, and workforce shortages. Chaos theory requires the system to allow for ambiguity and experimentation in directing changes to a positive outcome. An organization must be flexible to adapt to everyday situations. Collaboration of all parts of the system to continuous problem solving must occur in a complex organization that prioritizes the changes needed.

Complexity Theory

Complexity theory has its origins from the chaos model, in which changes are rapid, random, and frequent. Organizations in health care are complex and reflect individual characteristics as well as the mission/vision of the group and its leaders. Prior theories of organizations have viewed decision making from the top down. Current thought is that this idea is a narrow viewpoint that does not respond well to the rapidly changing healthcare environment. Complex organizations have many layers, resulting in a slow reaction to the change that is needed. Complexity theory allows for change at the point of care (POC) in a bottom-up scenario. The current trend is seen in hospitals aspiring to obtain Magnet recognition status awarded by the American Nurses Credentialing Center (ANCC). Decision making by the bedside nurse to change practice that is evidence-based is a classic example of how the nurse at the bedside can be a leader in a complex organization. The CNL using complexity theory at POC collaborates with peers and managers to achieve positive patient care outcomes. Complexity theory allows for concepts from many theories, collaborative relationships, and multiple solutions.

Dopson (2007) highlighted the work of Estabrook, who has extensively studied research leadership as it relates to organizational complexity. Translating research of organizational complexity into action requires the perspectives of process (not events), contesting knowledge (even random control trials), multiple stakeholders, and autonomy, to name a few. Dopson (2007) notes that Estabrook et al. see context as attitude, leadership, and decision making accomplished through macro, meso, and micro levels.

Within complex organizations, knowledge translation is a process grounded in real-life clinical settings. Boswell and Cannon (2007) stated, "Each nurse brings serviceable knowledge to the practice arena" (p. 4). Translating (using) research (evidence) at the POC by CNLs will result in new strategies for patient care that is not step by step or reactionary in delivery but rather an evolving process.

CNLs must be cognizant of leadership styles, change theories, and complexity to bring about change. As Dopson (2007) suggested in Estabrook's work, microsystems analysis needs to be considered because it is the POC where evidence is translated into practice.

Microsystem Analysis

According to Nelson et al. (2002, p. 473), "Clinical micro-systems are the small, functional, front-line units that provide most health care to most people." As any clinical microsystem is considered, the attributes and significance of the services provided within a large healthcare facility are interconnected to the care offered on any of the smaller units that make up the whole. Nelson et al. (2002, p. 473) stated that "a seamless, patient-centered, high-quality, safe, and efficient health system cannot be realized without the transformation of the essential building blocks that combine to form the care continuum." The individual parts must work effectively and efficiently together if the whole system is to be successful. King and Byers (2007) consider that healthcare professionals unconditionally look to the organizational traditions to determine the acceptable work models. The clinical microsystems are those essential elements that reflect the patterns of learning, adoption, and movement of knowledge and understanding within any agency. These indispensable units are the blood vessels within the organization that ensure that sustenance and life are enduring and profitable.

An essential and fundamental aspect within the leadership of any macrosystem must be the conscientious and meticulous examination of each microsystem. Linking micro- and macrosystems may move the facility toward a powerful and efficient institution. A reverse of this might be looking good on the outside, while being unproductive and destructive within. Nelson et al. (2002, p. 482) identified nine dimensions correlated to highly favorable systematic outcomes: "leadership; culture; macroorganization support of micro-systems; patient focus; staff focus; interdependence of care team; information and information technology; process improvement; and performance pattern." These nine characteristics flow from leading the organization to focus on the people, resulting in effective communication that triggers successful performance and improvement. As facets are analyzed and incorporated at the base units within an organization, the values of caring, listening, educating, and mentoring are reflected and integrated into the practical functioning of the individuals from the ground upward to the macrosystem. When the culture and involvement are effectively orchestrated at the most basic unit of the organization, a ripple effect occurs, resulting in a positive environment expansion from individuals at the bedside to the upper managerial levels.

According to King and Byers (2007, p. 21), "Organized efforts to promote a positive organizational culture, patient outcomes, and quality patient care are paramount." Emphasis on the achievement of successful, positive outcomes on the individual microsystem units demonstrates the straightforward attention to the individual and to the acceptable outcomes. Energy must be directed to "getting it right" at the basic level for the capacity for accomplishment and the intensity of realization to be reached. When healthcare systems revamp the strategic plan to bring about optimal performance at the bedside by exceeding patient and staff needs and expectations to address the vision and mission of the larger organization, transformation of the healthcare environment ensues. Watkins, Jones, and Norman (2006, p. 13) note that "nurse leaders must be able to demonstrate a sophisticated comprehension of the organization and political context in which they work and to tailor their leadership styles accordingly." Nursing leaders functioning within the microsystem units must demonstrate the fundamental and essential characteristics of effective and innovative leaders committed to the advancement of the nursing profession.

Conclusions

The CNL faces opportunities and challenges in providing patient care in the healthcare arena today and in the future. The first opportunity for the CNL is to select a primary leadership style and identify the style of the partnering nurse manager in the area assigned. These should be complementary in order to facilitate change directed at quality and safe care delivery and the development of staff as lifelong learners. Finding a traditional or nontraditional style must reflect individual characteristics of the CNL. Leaders must be comfortable in their style to be effective in moving members of the healthcare team toward a common goal. Even when having a predominant leadership style, CNLs must realize that at times, given unique situations, any of the traditional or nontraditional styles could be used to maximize the success for a given critical challenge. As a result, CNLs must understand the different styles when the strengths of one style may be needed to confront and manage a particular situation.

Once a style of leadership is understood, the CNL seeks to better understand change theory. Regardless of whether change is planned or unplanned, change is a constant in health care. Planned change occurs in incremental steps, whereas unplanned change creates complexity and sometimes chaos. According to Hendel, Fish, and Berger (2007), current organizational characteristics command that individuals engage in conversations reflective of ideas and approaches that can be contradictory while requiring coordination, negotiation, and/or collaboration. Complex organizations require the CNL to be cognizant of leadership styles, change theories, and complexity science. In addition, microsystem analysis is essential to the provision of clinical services at the bedside. The challenge for the CNL is to fit all the pieces together when leading and managing care at the bedside. As Grossman and Valiga (2009) indicated, we can all be leaders to move the profession forward and make a difference in the future.

Tools of the Trade: Case Studies

Case Study 1: Assignment as a Clinical Nurse Leader

You have been employed as a CNL on a medical-surgical unit. This unit has been under the direction of an experienced RN who has held the nurse manager (NM) position for over 10 years. The NM is well liked on the unit. The chief nursing officer does not consider the functioning of the unit to be appropriate due to frequent demands for more help, lack of discipline and accountability, complaints from patient families, and difficulty voiced by individuals floated to the unit. The core staff members do not want a change in leadership. They are comfortable with the current leadership and how the unit operates, and have not been educated on the CNL role and the advantages.

Consider the following questions related to this scenario:

1. What type of leadership style would you consider using with this situation, and why?
2. Which of the change theories do you envision using to help make the changes required for this unit?
3. Discuss key aspects that will need to be queried within a microsystem analysis of this unit. Why these aspects?

4. What strategies and techniques will you use to educate the staff on the CNL role and advantages in order to have a successful impact?

Case Study 2: Hospital Takeover by a "For-Profit" Company

The hospital where you work as a CNL has recently been bought by a "for-profit" company from out of state. The new management is beginning the assessment phase for assuming the management of the agency. The staff on your unit is worried about the upcoming changes and the impact they will have on maintaining the CNL position because the new owners have not historically employed CNLs.

Consider the following questions related to this scenario:

1. What type of activities can the CNL and nurse manager use to reduce the stress and worry currently encountered on your unit?
2. What leadership style would best serve to sustain and advance the unit during this process, and why?
3. What type of microsystem analysis would your unit document to reflect its quality and experience for review by the incoming management agency?

Case Study 3: Achieving Magnet Status

The institution where you are working as a CNL has decided to begin a Magnet journey within ANCC. The nursing administration team has determined that unit practice councils will be established to engage the staff nurse within the department decision-making process. You have been given the directive to organize and facilitate the unit practice council for the nursing unit on which you work.

Consider the following questions related to this scenario:

1. What leadership style would be employed in this situation to advance the acceptance of the unit practice council plan?
2. What issues related to change do you anticipate having to address? How do you plan to confront and address these issues?

Summary

- Leadership requires a leader who is able to use tasks, skills, and abilities to move a plan forward toward successful completion.
- The development of the CNL is of paramount importance as expert leaders currently navigating the complex healthcare delivery environment begin to leave the work environment. This departure of the skilled leaders will leave a void in the nursing leadership ranks if CNLs are not mentored and developed as this critical changeover proceeds.
- The three traditional leadership styles are designated as autocratic, democratic, and laissez-faire.
- Succession planning with the growing crises in nursing must be embraced to allow for organizational continuity, which should secure tactical and operational efficacy.
- An effective leader is driven to develop and support each member of the group as he or she grows into his or her highest potential for success within the nursing profession.
- Collaboration of all parts of the system to continuous problem solving must occur in a complex organization that prioritizes the necessary changes.
- As any clinical microsystem is considered, the attributes and significance of the services provided within a large healthcare facility are interconnected to the care offered on any of the smaller units that make up the whole.
- The clinical microsystems are those essential elements that reflect the patterns of learning, adoption, and movement of knowledge and understanding within any agency.

Reflection Questions

1. What types of leadership styles have you worked within an employment setting? Which of these styles are you the most comfortable with engaging in, and why?
2. Looking at your healthcare facility, identify the different microsystem components. What are some of the strengths and weaknesses of these different components?

Learning Activities

1. Interview the chief nursing officer within your organization to determine what types of succession planning are occurring within the institution. What plans are in place to prepare the next generation of leaders, including CNLs, within your organization?

2. Follow a change initiative of the system in which you are involved in your CNL immersion experience. How would you describe the change process? Is it as effective as it could be? How is this measured? Identify barriers to the change process. What "theories in action" are you not observing as you work through the process?

References

American Association of Colleges of Nursing (AACN). (2007). *White paper on the education and role of the clinical nurse leader.* Washington, DC: Author.

Barnhart, C. L., & Stein, J. (Eds.). (1962). *The American college dictionary.* New York: Random House.

Beyers, M., (2006, June). Nurse executives' perspectives on succession planning. *Journal of Nursing Administration, 36*(6), 304–312.

Boswell, C., & Cannon, S. (2007). *Introduction to nursing research: Incorporating evidence-based practice.* Sudbury, MA: Jones and Bartlett.

Dopson, S. (2007). A view from organization studies. *Nursing Research, 56*(4), 72–77.

Estabrooks, C. A. (1997). *Research utilization in nursing: An examination of formal structure and influencing factors.* Unpublished doctoral dissertation, University of Alberta, Edmonton, Alberta.

Estabrooks, C. A., Field, P. A., & Morse, J. M. (1994). Aggregating qualitative findings: An approach to theory development. *Qualitative Health Research, 4*(4), 503–511.

Grossman, S. C., & Valiga, T. M. (2009). *The new leadership challenge: Creating the future of nursing* (3rd ed.). Philadelphia: F.A. Davis.

Hartranft, S. R., Garcia, T., & Adams, N. (2007, June). Realizing the anticipated effects of the clinical nurse leader. *Journal of Nursing Administration, 37*(6), 261–263.

Havilock, R. G. (1973). *The change agent's guide to innovation in education.* Englewood Cliffs, NJ: Educational Technology Publications.

Hendel, T., Fish, M., & Berger, O. (2007, July/September). Nurse/physician conflict management mode choices: Implications for improved collaborative practice. *Nursing Administration Quarterly, 31*(3), 244–253.

Jooste, K. D. (2004, May). Leadership: A new perspective. *Journal of Nursing Management, 12*(3), 217–223.

King, T., & Byers, J. F. (2007, January). A review of organization culture instruments for nurse executives. *Journal of Nursing Administration, 37*(1), 21–31.

Lewin, K. (1947). Frontiers in group dynamics: Concepts, methods, and reality in social science, social equilibrium and social changes. *Human Relations, 1*(1), 5–41.

Lippit, R., Watson, J., & Westley, B. (1958). *The dynamics of planned change.* New York: Harcourt Brace.

Longest, B. B. (2004). *Managing health programs and projects.* San Francisco: Jossey-Bass.

Morgan, D. A., Johnson, J. G., & Garrison, D. R. (2007). Nurses leading change. In R. A. Patronis Jones (Ed.), *Nursing leadership and management theories, processes, and practice* (pp. 167–182). Philadelphia: F. A. Davis.

Nelson, E. C., Batalden, P. B., Huber, T. P., Mohr, J. J., Godfrey, M. M., Headrick, L. A., et al. (2002). Microsystems in health care: Part 1. Learning from high-performing front-line clinical unit. *Joint Commission Journal on Quality Improvement, 28*(9), 472–493.

Peck, D. (2007, August). Leadership development through self-awareness. *Talent Management.* Retrieved August 27, 2007, from http://www.talentmgt.com/learning_development/2007/August/393/index.php

Rogers, E. (1983). *Diffusion of innovations.* New York: Free Press.

Senge, P. M. (1990). *The fifth discipline: The art and practice of learning organizations.* New York: Doubleday.

Thies, K. M., & Ayers, L. (2007, July). Academic microsystems: Adapting clinical microsystems as an evaluation framework for community-based nursing education. *Journal of Nursing Education, 46*(7), 325–328.

Watkins, M., Jones, R., & Norman, S. (2006, December). Good care is good business. *Nursing Management, 13*(8), 12–14.

Webster's II new college dictionary. (1999). Boston: Houghton Mifflin.

Yoder-Wise, P. S. (2007). *Leading and managing in nursing* (4th ed.). St. Louis, MO: Elsevier/Mosby.

Yoder-Wise, P. S., & Kowalski, K. E. (2006). *Beyond leading and managing: Nursing administration for the future.* St. Louis, MO: Mosby.

SIX

Effective Communication and Team Coordination

■ **Deborah Antai-Otong**

■ Learning Objectives

- ■ Explore the concept of effective use of self as related to written and verbal communication, interpersonal relations, diversity, ethical principles, and professional nursing.
- ■ Discuss the management of the health-care environment through the concepts

> "The way we feel about ourselves is often communicated by the way we treat others."
>
> Anonymous

of delegation and supervision, interdisciplinary care coordination, group dynamics, and conflict resolution.

Key Terms

Assertiveness
Coalition and team building
Communication
Conflict

Group dynamics
Organizational trust
Team

CNL Roles

Clinician
Client advocate
Information manager
Team manager

Outcome manager
Educator
Lifelong learner
Member of a profession

CNL Professional Values

Altruism
Human dignity

Accountability
Integrity

CNL Core Competencies

Critical thinking
Illness and disease management
Ethics
Healthcare systems and policy
Designer/manager/coordinator of care
Communication

Information and healthcare technologies
Human diversity
Provider and manager of care
Nursing technology and resource
   management

Introduction

Role of the Beginning CNL: Clinician and Team Leader

The beginning clinical nurse leader (CNL) has opportunities to implement evidence-based care across the healthcare continuum. The success of this role delineation is based on effective communication skills and interpersonal relations that advance patient-centered care. Successful deployment also requires a basic understanding of human interactions, communication, problem-solving skills, conflict management, and coalition or team building.

The quality of all relationships stems from effective communication and concerns, and appreciation of the rights and respect for others. Effective communication is the matrix of nursing and a critical tool for the CNL regardless of practice setting or role. This is particularly significant in an era of vast technological advances and substantial reliance on nonverbal communication interactions, such as e-mails, faxes, blog entries, and tweets, to convey, interpret, and transmit messages.

Technological advances are increasingly changing the way consumers and providers communicate and deliver care. The impact of this trend continues to transform the manner in which healthcare services are crafted, planned, and delivered, and the course of nurse-patient interactions. Increasingly, consumers are communicating with their providers through the Internet and providers are communicating electronically with each other, insurance companies, and other entities. Data from electronic records can be collected, trended, and used to track treatment outcomes and improve care.

Telecommunication also expands the range of tools with which people communicate—from microphone, camera, loudspeaker, cell phones, and Internet to rapidly emerging personal hardware, including cell phones with cameras, iPods, MP3 players, and Skype.

In general, information technologies are an integral part of our lives and invaluable in many instances because information and communication are immediate and easily accessed. Immediate access is cost effective and time efficient. Despite these advantages and efficiency, however, telecommunications may thwart the natural process of human encounters. The beginning CNL is challenged to balance advantages and disadvantages and to design innovative communication processes that facilitates and sustain quality interpersonal relationships. (Chapter 9 provides an in-depth discussion of informatics and technology).

Although the healthcare arena excels in trending and improving quality of care, consumers, both internal and external, are more interested in processes and who delivers services. Accordingly, advances in technology focus primarily on values and objectivity of science, with little emphasis on individual preferences, needs, values, and preferences. Healthy human interactions provide a venue for the CNL to form quality interpersonal relationships through effective communication to address and resolve the needs of consumers and to implement evidence-based interventions and develop and improve across the healthcare continuum.

This chapter focuses on the effective use of self as related to effective communication, interpersonal relations, ethical principles, and professional values. The initial discussion focuses on essential qualities in the CNL—the foundation of communication, interpersonal relationships, and professional values. Latter discussion integrates these principles into leadership skills and management of healthcare environments through delegation, supervision, interdisciplinary coordination of care, team building, group dynamics, and conflict management.

Essential Qualities of the Clinical Nurse Leader

Regardless of where clinical nurse leaders enter healthcare systems, they must possess essential qualities or competencies that enable them to quickly establish meaningful relationships and to work effectively as a leader, team member, team leader, and broker of health care across the healthcare continuum. Essential qualities are shaped by age, culture, gender, ethnicity, and educational and socioeconomic factors. These factors must be considered when conversing with internal and external consumers to ensure that verbal and nonverbal communication is appropriately transmitted and received.

Essential qualities, or core competencies, are the building blocks of effective communication and interpersonal relationships. Essential qualities are therapeutic use of self, genuineness, warmth, empathy, acceptance, maturity, and self-awareness (Antai-Otong, 2008). Each quality promotes respect, maintains human dignity, displays care and acceptance, and sustains healthy interpersonal relations.

1. *Therapeutic use of self* is a core quality of nursing. It engenders trust and acceptance and a willingness to share personal experiences. Sharing personal feelings helps the nurse glean insight into another person's experience. This interactive process requires active listening skills, such as attentiveness and patience, congruent verbal and nonverbal communication, and mutual respect. It allows the CNL to impart

support, reassurance, and health education, and to gather important data collection to ensure appropriate decision making.

2. *Genuineness* refers to honesty and authenticity and infers openness and lack of defensiveness. Genuineness and openness must be prudent, tactful, discreet, and appropriate. Genuineness is communicated verbally by the following comments: "This must be a difficult time for you. How can I assist?" Nonverbal communication occurs with a handshake, embrace (when appropriate), active listening, eye contact, and open body language such as unfolded or uncrossed legs. It is imperative that verbal and nonverbal communication are congruent when displaying genuineness.

3. *Warmth* is often associated with empathy, patience, kindness, and concerns for others. It may be expressed with a smile, handshake, or eye contact. Warmth and genuineness often occur simultaneously and are core elements of therapeutic use of self, quality interpersonal relations, high consumer confidence and satisfaction, and positive healthcare outcomes. A lack of warmth is perceived as "cold and aloof" and noncaring. It is likely to generate distrust, anger, resentment, poor treatment outcomes, and low consumer satisfaction.

4. *Empathy* is the capacity to identify with or vicariously experience another's situation, feelings, and motives without them becoming part of self. Its usefulness lies in helping the CNL "walk a mile in someone's shoes" and understanding the meaning of another's anger, sadness, joy, grief and other strong emotions. Empathy enables the CNL to use objective approaches to evaluate and resolve highly emotionally charged situations. It is the antithesis of pity, which infers one takes on the feelings and motives of others as one's own. Pity is counterproductive because it reduces objectivity and makes it difficult to separate one's feelings from others. It often leads to "rescuing" behaviors, blurred boundaries, and inappropriate relationships.

5. *Acceptance* refers to favorable reception, belief in or approval of others, and value of differences. The extent of acceptance arises from the individual's values, beliefs, maturity, nonjudgmental attitude or tolerance, and self-awareness. Rapid societal and demographic changes, particularly in race, age, ethnicity, gender, religious beliefs and health practices, necessitate greater value and appreciation, and acceptance of diversity and different views and attitudes. Inherent in acceptance is respect and maintenance of human dignity and integrity. For example, the CNL may encounter an emotionally charged situation in which a patient, family, or colleague is shouting. Although this behavior is unacceptable, the nurse must respond in an accepting manner using assertive and calming verbal and nonverbal communication to convey concern and willingness to help. The CNL must also quickly assess the problem and work

with the individual to resolve it in a timely manner, saying, for example, "I understand you are pretty upset because your prescription has not been filled, but is difficult to help if you are shouting. Let me check with pharmacy to see what has happened. I will be back in a few minutes." This approach involves therapeutic use of self, genuineness, warmth and caring, and acceptance, yet it is firm and calming.

6. *Maturity* extends beyond chronological age and entails the ease in which an individual forms trust and meaningful relationships, displays empathy and warmth, utilizes sound judgment, and demonstrates decision-making and problem-solving skills. Essential attributes of maturity include confidence in self and others, recognition of personal strengths and vulnerabilities, assertiveness, and overall respect for self and others. Individuals who lack these mature attributes tend to blame others for their mistakes, are argumentative and defensive, fail to see positives in others, and use manipulative behaviors to meet personal and professional needs. They tend to engender distrust and strong negative emotions in others and have difficulty forming trust and healthy interpersonal relations.

7. *Self-awareness* is governed by mature behaviors and involves acknowledging and understanding personal strengths and attributes, as well as shortcomings and vulnerabilities. Recognizing personal strengths and areas that require improvement helps the CNL appreciate these qualities in others. It promotes an objective portrait of how one fits into society within individual, groups, and organizational domains. It is imperative to understand oneself to form meaningful relationships, recognize and value personal and professional values, and negotiate with others. A lack of self-awareness often results in defensiveness, personalization of negative or constructive feedback, and unwillingness to listen to others and negotiate differences. The likely results are poor interpersonal relations, miscommunication, low consumer satisfaction, and poor outcomes.

In summary, the complexity of working with individuals, groups, and systems requires the CNL to acquire the aforementioned essential qualities. The successful CNL promotes self through effective communication skills, maintains personal balance, establishes coalitions across the healthcare continuum, and advances the values and mission of the organization. Predictably, distrust; impatience; failure to establish meaningful relationships and display empathy, warmth, and genuineness; and immature behaviors result in hostile work relationships, conflict, exhausted resources, and poor treatment outcomes.

As the beginning CNL understands self and uses essential qualities to work with others individually, in groups, and in organizations, personal and professional values will direct how they treat others, hold themselves accountable, and utilize sound judgment and decision making based on personal integrity and ethical principles. The following section describes these concepts and their impact on the CNL role.

Professional Values

The beginning CNL brings a repertoire of personal and professional values and beliefs based on innate attributes, knowledge, educational preparation, socioeconomic factors, and clinical expertise that either synchronizes with or diverges from organizational expectations, values, and beliefs. Divergence in values between staff and the organization often results in conflict and miscommunication, and may impact the successful deployment of the CNL role.

Professional values are individual and organizational expectations and ideas that direct social and environmental responsibilities, accountability, and proficiency. They influence decision making, communication, judgment, daily routines, and practices. These principles also underlie organizational policies, decision making and a culture that responds to internal and external consumers, and healthcare delivery (Lloyd, Wise, Weeramanthri, & Nugus, 2009).

Professional values—including *altruism, accountability and responsibility, human dignity, integrity*, and *ethical principles*—facilitate successful transition into the CNL role. Professional and personal values govern how we communicate; form interpersonal relations; respond to and manage conflicts; provide health care; respond to failure; view differences in others, including ethnicity and culture; cope with stress; accept success; and display empathy and concern for others.

Altruism is the practice or display of unselfish concern for or devotion to the welfare of others without regard to reward or benefits (Yalom & Leszcz, 2005). True altruism is natural and innate and occurs as a natural part of interactions with others. It is a character trait that is easily recognized and valued by others. The foundation of altruism is openness, empathy, genuineness, and sensitivity to the needs of others (Watson, 1988).

Accountability and responsibility are interrelated. Responsible people account for what they do, and how well they perform. They work effectively with others or individually and complete tasks and achieve expected outcomes. Accountability and responsibility generate trust that when you commit yourself, you will follow through to achieve the expected outcome. Trust is built on predictable behavior associated with keeping promises and being accountable even when expectations are not achieved.

It is a reliable way to build and sustain organizational trust, and it is a crucial leadership skill. Leadership skills are discussed later in this chapter.

Human dignity relates to our valuing of those we serve. It is the honor we give those we are privileged to care for in our daily work. It implies a respect for the uniqueness of one's culture and appreciation of diversity.

Integrity, an integral part of accountability and altruism, guides ethical decision making. It infers the individual consistently maintains and exhibits high character (e.g., follows societal and cultural norms, expectations, and professional standards). Strong integrity is directed by ethical principles and moral character. It also fosters trust, respect, personal confidence, and self-esteem.

Ethical principles and integrity are interrelated and comprise a moral framework in which the CNL frames practice. From a professional prospective, this includes a code of ethics to act according to the highest standards and mission of profession, conscience, and the organization. Principles of professional practice include integrity, honesty, truthfulness, and adherence to obligation to safeguard public trust. Ethical principles also include developing and maintaining professional knowledge and competencies to ensure performance, demonstrating concern for the well-being of others, adhering to all applicable federal and state and local laws and regulations, cultivating and valuing cultural diversity and pluralistic values, and treating all people with dignity and respect.

As the CNL role is deployed, its cost must be justified by healthcare organizations. The beginning CNL must seek employment prepared to lead with a vision guided by essential qualities, proficient communication skills, professional values, and a willingness to learn. He or she must quickly understand the mission, values, and expectations of the organization as demonstrated by results of external sources, such as The Joint Commission, care delivery models, safety history, clinical outcomes, and consumer and staff satisfaction. Lastly, the CNL must secure early wins and establish coalitions that produce organizational adjustments to environmental and political demands (Watkins, 2003). Most successful organizations value leadership as an asset and a sustainable competitive advantage. This advantage opens the door for the CNL, a natural leader, to be developed as a future leader.

Building Leadership Skills

Leadership is an integral part of nursing. The CNL has the advantage over some nurses because leadership is expected and encouraged. High-performing leaders make an impact on the success of the organization. They are expert communicators and coalition builders, and are culturally sensitive and proficient in technological advances. The transition from novice to expert leader evolves over time, but the aforementioned foundation facilitates leadership development.

The evolution of expert leadership skills requires confidence, a vision, and belief in oneself as a leader and contributor to the organization's values and mission. Normally, initial leadership roles generate tremendous anxiety and uncertainty. The CNL must employ effective communication and critical thinking skills, celebrate early successes, and nurture personal attributes to manage anxiety, uncertainties, and fears through constructive appraisal of self and others. High-functioning leaders use these building blocks to motivate individuals, groups, and systems toward a common goal. A positive, realistic, and confident attitude, coupled with core competencies in management and leadership, predicts success. Core competencies include *organizational trust, communication, problem solving and decision making, cultural sensitivity,* and *coalition building.*

Organizational Trust

Organizational trust is earned trust based on proven accountability, credibility, personal integrity, effective communication skills, and the ability to work with others and implement strategies with positive results. Trust, the heart of healthy relationships and effective communication, is not immediately granted to the beginning CNL. According to Barker (1992), organizational trust is not inherent and must be earned and nurtured through all encounters and situations. Organizational trust is rooted in role theory.

Role theory posits that members of the organization assume responsibilities and roles within the system (Biddle, 1986). Role expectations of a leader vary in scope. In one organization, the leader defines personal style; in another, roles are determined by organizational expectations held both by the individual and by other people. The beginning CNL must understand the role and expectations within the organization, including goals, actions, and outcomes along with performance and proficiency necessary in given situations or encounters. Trust arises from predictable behaviors based on actual or expected role performance. A substantial proportion of organizational trust is nurtured through observable, daily social interactions of individuals carrying out their roles.

Building trust involves an array of basic principles and behaviors. The CNL exhibits confidence and patience, employs effective communication skills, and validates expected technical proficiency as part of role development. Technical proficiency skills, such as data management and computer literacy, are critical competencies for the CNL. In addition, the CNL must do the following:

- Demonstrate knowledge and clinical competency about the subject matter;
- Ask appropriate questions and seek advice from mentor;
- Keep promises, establish realistic and measureable outcomes, and meet deadlines;
- Seek to understand others' positions;
- Employ assertive communication skills;
- Exhibit consistency and reliability;
- Express genuine interest and enthusiasm about the subject matter;
- Accept other's feelings and ideas, which does not mean you agree;
- Encourage active participation in decision making;
- Provide ongoing feedback using an assertive and constructive approach;
- Recognize and celebrate strengths and successes;
- Recognize vulnerabilities; and
- Be accountable for failures and vulnerabilities, and learn from these experiences.

Every encounter and situation, positive and negative, is an opportunity to learn and grow. Growth from these experiences occurs with time and is based on understanding nurse leaders' roles and expectations. Increasing evidence implicates strong leadership skills as necessary to work effectively with others, advance the mission and values of the organization, and facilitate positive outcomes.

Early successes require CNLs to identify and resolve organizational barriers inherent in their roles and implementation of evidence-based practice. Of particular interest are a lack of time, inadequate resources, a lack of nursing autonomy and empowerment, and cultural factors. Growing evidence demonstrates significant correlations between these barriers and practice, knowledge, and attitudes associated with evidence-based practice. Solutions to overcome these barriers include learning opportunities, mentoring, culture and relationship building, and cost-effective outcomes (Brown, Wickline, Ecoff, & Glaser, 2009; Koehn & Lehman, 2008).

A qualitative study that focused primarily on performance of the nurse consultant's role in relation to the transformational leadership theory concluded that participants ($n = 4$) lacked considerable technical competencies, cognitive and interpersonal skills, and risk taking (McIntosh & Tolson, 2009). As a result of early findings from the study, leadership implemented several approaches to facilitate transformational leadership skills and processes that included developing a vision for designated services, acting as mentors and champions, and using assertive communication and interpersonal skills to advance complex change initiatives. They emphasized the importance of organizational support and educational opportunities to develop effective communication, and interpersonal skills that facilitate role development and competencies to attain outcomes (McIntosh & Tolson, 2009).

Organizational trust is also guided by unique contributions of the CNL, particularly leading research-driven activities and practice. Integration of research into clinical nursing practice is pivotal in the delivery of high-quality health care (Cummings, Estabrooks, Midodzi, Wallin, & Hayduk, 2007; Kajermo et al., 2008). CNLs must integrate research findings into practice. This can be attained by making their practice more research transparent by providing necessary leadership, enlisting staff participation at all levels within the organization, establishing a research agenda, and implementing evidence-based practice to improve outcomes. Although CNLs, along with other staff, are not provided ample time to lead research-driven research activities and lack motivation to review studies and apply findings to practice, it is critical to consider these initiatives to promote organizational trust and improve outcomes (Chummun & Tiran, 2008). Conclusions from this study indicate that successful organizational trust requires effective communication and interpersonal skills, confidence and patience, and clinical competencies to lead and participate in complex situations and encounters.

High-performing leaders clearly understand the significance of purpose, vision, and alignment to revitalizing the organization. Leaders must discern what drives organizational success and expectations. What does the organization expect about health care, internal and external consumers, quality, and safety? Are providers expected to develop and implement evidence-based interventions and clinical outcomes? What healthcare models are in place to address and manage complex patient problems and ensure appropriate monitoring, tracking, and trending quality improvement activities? Does the organization embrace evidence-based practice? If not, why? By answering these questions, the CNL can generate ideas and develop a niche within the organization that is consistent with its mission, values, and expectations. How can this knowledge guide the CNL to lead an initiative that facilitates implementation of evidence-based practice? How can leadership skills be used to initiate this practice on one unit, additional units, and ultimately the entire organization? Successful implementation of the team and later positive outcomes demonstrate how the CNL can create opportunities to lead activities by engaging others through coalition building and establish positive outcomes.

High-performing leaders are astute and proficient communicators who advance the mission and values of the organization and develop personal and professional goals. Clearly, organizational trust is built on and driven by effective communication.

Communication

A fundamental part of our daily lives, communication occurs within vast encounters and situations. It is the transmission of feelings, attitudes, ideas, and behaviors between people. It is complex and involves numerous components, including verbal and nonverbal exchanges, active listening, assertiveness, conflict management, and communication issues unique to individuals and situations.

Maxwell (1999) describes four essential qualities of effective communicators:

- *Convey a Clear and Simple Message*: Communication extends beyond what is said and includes how the message is delivered. Keeping it simple helps you connect with others.
- *See the Whole Person*: Convey respect and belief in others. Use active listening skills.
- *Show the Truth*: Display confidence, and believe in what you say. Demonstrate credibility.
- *Seek a Response*: Clarify so that the correct message is communicated. The goal of communication is action: give the recipient something to feel, think, remember, and do, and motivate others.

In today's rapidly changing world, communication is likely to be transmitted via technology rather than face to face. More and more people are communicating through text message, e-mail, conference call, and phone or video conference. Regardless of the venue, communication occurs at many levels and requires skills that facilitate healthy work relationships, impart information, convey respect, and address consumer and organizational needs. An inconsiderate message or response via e-mail may be more damaging to a relationship than simply picking up the phone to call after abating one's anger or frustration. Technology takes away the human component of feelings, warmth, and eye contact and leaves the sender and recipient to decipher words rather than verbal and nonverbal cues. In contrast, face-to-face interactions provide a forum for body language and verbal communication to convey a

Table 6-1   Giving and Receiving Feedback

- Clearly state what you want to say.
- Emphasize the positive.
- Be specific.
- Focus on the behavior rather than the person.
- Refer to behavior that can be changed.
- Be descriptive rather than evaluative.
- Use "I" statements rather than "you" statements to reduce defensiveness.
- Avoid using generalizations such as "always" or "never."
- Avoid giving advice.

message. Verbal and nonverbal communication based on mutual understanding and respect is necessary as the CNL expects to support individuals, families, colleagues, and organizations.

Intrinsically, nurses are confronted with the daily challenge of deciphering others' verbal and nonverbal messages and responses. Communication enables the CNL to realize the complexity of human interactions and form meaningful relationships with others. Whether interacting with the patient or family at the bedside or among a group of colleagues or presenting data to senior leadership, the CNL must command effective communication skills and use verbal and nonverbal cues to convey clear messages and respond to others appropriately. Both qualitative and quantitative studies have presented evidence of the benefits of effective communication, particularly in critical care settings (Engström & Söderberg, 2007; O'Connell & Landers, 2008).

Communication styles are influenced by individual differences, which include developmental stage, gender, socioeconomic factors, values, religion, health practices, psychosocial factors, culture, ethnicity, and language. Changing societal demographics play a critical role in how messages are communicated and deciphered. These changes require nurse leaders to recognize personal attributes, beliefs and values, and differences in others when communicating with others. A common communication error is a failure to listen and trying to read others' minds or expecting them to read ours. In order for others to respond to our needs and ideas, we must clearly communicate what they are and convey them in a manner that others can understand and respond appropriately (see Table 6-1).

Body language, or nonverbal communication, such as tone of voice, sweat on the brow or palms, dress, hygiene, facial expression, posture, and gait can also be misinterpreted. Nonverbal communication must be clarified when in doubt to ensure accurate interpretation of the message. Verbal and nonverbal messages must be congruent. For instance, if your voice tone is loud and your speech is rapid, one may conclude that you are anxious or angry. If confronted about "anger," it is imperative to assess how messages are being conveyed rather than being defensive. The more congruent the nonverbal cues are with the verbal, the clearer the message. This is particularly important when communicating highly charged, controversial, or important results, issues, or requests.

Verbal communication involves an exchange of words, both spoken and written, between people. One cannot assume that what is spoken and/or written is understood by the recipient of the message. It is imperative to look for verbal and nonverbal cues that ensure the correct message is heard and understood. Verbal communication requires the following (Antai-Otong, 2008):

- An unhurried and confident approach;
- Knowledge and preparation of subject matter;
- Good eye contact;
- Adequate personal space: ample distance between self and others;
- Assertive posture;
- Simple, clear explanations based on education, developmental stage, gender, culture, ethnicity, and cognitive function; and
- Active listening skills.

Active listening is interactive and requires full attention, notably suspending multitasking or other activities; it includes appropriate verbal and nonverbal cues, such as nods, forward movement, and appropriate responses. Body language, or nonverbal communication, defines whether the recipient is actively listening. Allow the person speaking to complete sentences and train of thought without interruptions. This is critical to fully hearing the speaker's point of view or processing information, while demonstrating respect. An effective listener concentrates and mentally summarizes content (sender's main points), listens for themes or central point, analyzes the evidence, and integrates it into the communication process and responds accordingly. Confirmation that the message is clearly understood can be conveyed by paraphrasing, restating the central idea, or by asking a question that conveys understanding of the main idea. These techniques are an excellent method to check or validate assumptions about nonverbal and verbal communication. Lastly, an easy way to remember relevant or salient points of a message exchange is to recollect an encounter or situation in which you felt at ease and comfortable, and heard and conveyed feelings, thoughts, and issues that concerned you. What put you at ease—the person and/or the environment? The following points reinforce techniques useful in active listening:

- Use of self when making salient points;
- Genuineness;
- Warmth and acceptance;
- Shared values; and
- Assurance in your ability to solve your problem.

Consider these factors during your next encounter. Self-awareness is critical to how we listen to and communicate with others. Active listening is the heart of effective communication. The active listener is reflective, empathetic, and nonjudgmental, and avoids blurring issues with guilt or put-down statements.

A poor listener is inattentive, lacks warmth or "connectedness" with the sender, and uses encounters and situations to advance personal agenda or values. Poor listening skills, incongruent verbal and nonverbal cues, a failure to use active listening skills, and a lack of interest in the encounter or situation cause *miscommunication*. It is costly, nonproductive, and it reduces work productivity and consumer satisfaction. Miscommunication is also associated with passive and aggressive communication skills. Effective leaders use assertive communication skills.

Assertive communication is based on the premise that everyone has a right to meet their own needs, believe in themselves, and express feelings, thoughts, and ideas with mutual respect for others. Assertiveness is learned and difficult for some people. High self-esteem and self-worth, self-awareness, and confidence are the matrix of assertiveness. It is not only the message that distinguishes assertiveness, even though words must be carefully crafted, but it is also nonverbal communication and congruence with verbal communication that constitutes this communication skill.

Stress impacts how messages are received and heard. Normally, high emotional states or stressful situations interfere with what one hears and interprets from the sender. Reduced attention is linked to stress and high anxiety and tension. It is critical that individuals control their anxiety or stress by using deep breathing exercises to reduce their heart rate and respiration to reduce stress reactions. Thoughts are clearer and more focused when anxiety levels decrease. A failure to manage stress reactions results in ineffective verbal and nonverbal communication manifested by yelling, sharp or curt responses, and the inability to convey messages in a clear and

Table 6-2   Assertive Communication Techniques

- Control anger and strong emotions through deep breathing exercises or other stress reduction measures.
- Use a firm yet friendly and confident voice tone.
- Use nonthreatening body language including eye contact (consider cultural factors and appropriate distance—usually leg's length).
- Be specific.
- State what you mean: "I am concerned that every time we are in staff meeting you ignore me when I ask a question," "When you ignore me, I feel angry and insulted," or "In the future, when I ask a question I would appreciate it if you respond or answer my questions."
- Own your feelings, thoughts, and ideas (use "I" statements).
- Use active listening skills.
- Allow the other person to complete sentence or thoughts.
- Display respect.

respectful manner. Yelling, shouting, and angry responses often produce the same negative response in others. Assertive communication affords the following benefits:

- Enhances self-esteem and confidence;
- Facilitates respect;
- Reduces stress and anxiety;
- Promotes overall health;
- Allows one to say "no" without guilt;
- Helps parties state ideas, thoughts, and feelings more clearly;
- Allows expression of feelings, thoughts, and ideas without the intent of provoking others;
- Engenders open and honest communication and mutual respect; and
- Promotes win-win outcomes (see Table 6-2).

All in all, communication is an integral part of our lives. Its effectiveness is multifaceted and guided by mutual respect between parties, assertiveness skills, verbal and nonverbal communications, cultural factors and self-awareness, confidence, and self-esteem. It promotes quality and healthy interpersonal relationships that are rich, genuine, honest, and open. Effective communication skills require constant fine-tuning to ensure that we convey thoughts and ideas in a respectful and clear manner

Table 6-3   Comparison of Assertive, Passive, and Aggressive Communication

Assertive	Passive	Aggressive
Confident, self-respecting, goal oriented	Puts other's needs above own	Puts personal needs over others' with intent to intimidate, manipulate, demean, and threaten
Active listening	Low self-esteem	
A choice	Uses demeaning body language	
Open and honest		Manipulative
Direct	Low voice tone	Angry
Trusting	Lacks confidence	Vengeful
Focuses on unacceptable behavior and not the person	Helplessness	Distrustful
	Distrustful	Focus on other—blame
	Angry at self and others	Defensive and resentful
Based on mutual respect and meeting personal needs without compromising others' needs	Afraid to hurt others' feelings	Loud and threatening body language, intrusive
	Anxious demeanor	
	Poor eye contact	
Requires congruent body language, such as normal voice tone, eye contact, and appropriate distance	Lack of self-respect	Righteous, derogatory
	Guilt-driven decision making	Win-lose position (win at all costs and at the expense of others)
Win-win positions	Lose-win positions	

to advance health care using problem-solving and decision-making skills that produce positive outcomes (see Table 6-3).

Problem Solving and Decision Making

Much of what clinical nurse leaders do involves problem solving and decision making, as defined by professional and personal values, the organization, and consumers. It is imperative to involve the right people in the planning and implementation process. A natural reaction to problems is a quick and reactive response, but some problems and decisions are not easily solved and require additional time and resources. Several guidelines can facilitate this process:

- Define the problem with input from internal and external consumers, major stakeholders, and leadership. Evaluate complex problems, and avoid being overwhelmed or intimidated by closely scrutinizing the real problem.
- Evaluate underlying causes of the problem, and seek opinions or input from others. This may occur within various venues using diverse approaches, including brainstorming and prioritizing the problems.
- Explore options based on priorities, required resources, input from others, and timelines.
- Determine an approach.
- Develop a plan of action that includes the following:
  a. Measurable, realistic, and attainable goals
  b. Strategies or activities
  c. Objectives
  d. Responsible person(s)
  e. Resources/budget
- Implement plan.
- Monitor progress based on identified problems, resources, responsible person(s), and timelines.

In conclusion, problem solving and decision making occur at all levels within the organization. The CNL is instrumental in seeking input from key team members, internal and external consumers, and stakeholders to ensure that relevant information and resources are used to implement action plans, trend and track data and outcomes, and resolve problems.

Cultural Sensitivity

This leadership quality is an integral part of all encounters and situations. It influences organizational trust, communication, and problem solving. The complexity of cultural sensitivity requires a lengthier discussion that this chapter allows. However, multiple considerations are used to guide implementation, such as race, ethnicity, gender, religion, health practices, culture, language, sexual orientation, socioeconomic status, educational preparation, and country and region of origin. No approach fits all encounters or situations. Cultural sensitivity infers individualized approaches that ensure respect, acceptance, and tolerance consistent with individual wishes, preferences, beliefs, and values. These qualities are inherent in healthy interpersonal relationships and must be considered within social contexts and treatment planning for both patients and providers.

Coalition Building: An Essential Competency for the CNL

Consensus is emerging that integrated delivery systems provide strong support to the CNL integrated care coordination teams, offering patients great promise for improving quality and reducing costs (Scheetz, Bolon, Postelnick, Noskin, & Lee, 2009). Effective teams are based on effective communication and team-building skills, membership, and group dynamics.

Team Building

Team building involves developmental stages and processes to improve mutual performance. Similar to interpersonal relations, it evolves over time and requires necessary people and resources to facilitate organizational changes and outcomes. The effectiveness and efficiency of teams is determined by the purpose of the team, team member composition, and participation. The role of the CNL in team formation ranges from informal to formal and is based on individual and organizational needs. Research indicates that teams provide an invaluable contribution to the organization.

Strategies to establish and maintain team building fall into four domains:

1. *Personal competencies*: develop individual competencies; establish understand shared processes.
2. *Interpersonal skills*: improve group dynamics; engender common purpose and commitment.
3. *Organizational structure*: resolve barriers between various services within the organization (e.g., turf issues).
4. *Organizational environment*: build a team with distinguishing characteristics within the larger organization.

Successful team building requires four essential qualities: trust, open and effective communication, member involvement, and clearly defined measurable goals/outcomes (Antai-Otong, 1997). Effective teams require appropriate member selection based on a willingness to participate, confidence, proven history of following through on previous committees or teams, and mastery of effective communication skills. The CNL must be competent to lead and participate as a team member and model these behaviors in various situations and encounters.

An important feature of successful team building, *member involvement*, is a sense of commitment to the team, respect for team members, and enthusiasm for understanding team dynamics. Involved members value diversity, genuineness, and open-mindedness; display empathy; and are emotionally invested in the team and goal attainment. Team members feel linked to the larger system and are willing to collaborate and negotiate with others. Although they value their own role and contributions to the team, they perceive themselves as part of the whole, with the intent to reach common goals (Antai-Otong, 1997).

A *team* is a group that works toward a single, common goal, although members might have diverse individual goals. Teams can be informal or formal and include members from various parts of the healthcare system. Interdisciplinary teams and care planning are commonly found in specialty areas and are required to meet Joint Commission and other national standards involving healthcare issues. These teams often include professionals from various disciplines, patients, their families, and/or significant others and stakeholders (Meltzer et al., 2009).

On the whole, team members possess vast technical skills and clinical expertise and are encouraged to develop new ones that foster their versatility, adaptability, and value to the overall team. Team members are responsible for monitoring, trending, and tracking the overall process of goal attainment along with delegating problem-solving tasks to members. Successful teams foster trust, creativity, and risk taking by allowing members to listen and share their thoughts and feelings without being reprimanded (Attaran & Nguyen, 1999). Despite individual goals, the team's goals advance the higher collective one. For example, one Joint Commission team may track and trend tracers, another might conduct tracers, and yet another may participate on the Quality Executive Council. Yet all are accountable for preparation of a successful Joint Commission survey. Growing empirical data indicate positive clinical outcomes associated with self-directed teams. In a time of reduced resources, complex healthcare issues, and emphasis on positive clinical outcomes, teams provide a cost-effective approach to advance implementation rates of proven safety outcomes (Krimsky et al., 2009).

Team Selection

The success of team and coalition building originates in the selection process. Coalition and team building involves consolidating existing supporting, established relationships among key players; aligning self with persons in positions of power; and mobilizing resources. The novice CNL must assess where power lies in the organization and align him- or herself with persons in positions of power. He or she should observe how these individuals conduct meetings, respond to differences, and manage and control resources. Equally important is identification of mentors or individuals who are supportive, resourceful, and knowledgeable about navigating power and exerting influence within the organization. Influential people in the organization are critical resources for the CNL and provide the following resources (Watkins, 2003):

- *Expertise*: knowledge, experience, competencies;
- *Access to information*: information technology, computers, software;
- *Status*: level of power and influence in the organization;
- *Capital*: budgets, resources, and finances; and
- *Loyalty*: trust, reliability, and support.

Watkins (2003) also describes the following steps to coalition building:

- *Map the influence landscape.* A common mistake among new leaders is spending excessive time during transition within the vertical dimension of influence (e.g., supervisor, senior leadership) rather than the horizontal dimension (e.g., colleagues, peers). The most basic relationships must occur within horizontal dimensions, among colleagues, interdisciplinary groups, and consumers. These relationships are more likely to yield early successes and build the infrastructure for vertical areas in the organization.

- *Identify key players.* Team composition is critical to effective problem identification, decision making, planning, and outcomes. Involve internal and external team members, consumers, and stakeholders during early coalition building. Considerations for member selection should be guided by individual strengths, education, expertise in a given area, and whether they support professional and organizational values. Ground rules about behaviors, accountability, responsibility, and interpersonal and communication skills reduce the time required to create and sustain group cohesiveness. Group cohesiveness is widely researched and a basic component of groups. It generates a sense of "*we*-ness," supports common values and greater solidarity, protects against internal and external threats, and provides mutual support (Yalom & Leszcz, 2005).

- *List supporters and opponents.* Supporters share your vision for the future, values, and mutual respect for professional and organizational goals. They are change agents with demonstrated effective interpersonal skills and team-oriented results. Normally, opponents object to you no matter what, resisting changes and rejecting your vision for the future. They perceive team goals as a threat to their influence or power, values, and goals. Oftentimes they are the "informal leaders" who exert power at the grassroots or unit level. Engaging opponents in the coalition-building process is critical to garner their buy-in through healthy interpersonal interactions, which minimizes energy used to address push-back and resistance.

■ *Use tools of persuasion.* These are generally effective communication skills, especially assertiveness and the ability to influence and create alliances within the organization (Watkins, 2003). It is imperative to use these tools to garner influence, increase your visibility and credibility across the healthcare continuum, and open doors, such as getting an agenda on various committees. As the CNL navigates within various aspects of the healthcare continuum, it is imperative to understand the principles and value of group dynamics.

Common mistakes made by the beginning CNL as team member or leader is delay in reaching expected outcomes within designated timelines due to poor planning, unrealistic goals, inappropriate membership, inadequate resources and organizational support, and lack knowledge about group dynamics. To mitigate these mistakes, it is important to assess the organizational alignment with the team and use this to guide decision making, planning, and implementation. Strategies to achieve these goals include the following questions:

1. What is the team's alignment with organizational values, goals, and outcomes?
2. What decisions are required to ensure that team goals, implementation, timelines, and outcomes are consistent with the organization's goals, mission, and values?
3. What is the game plan to meet mutual goals?
4. How do we implement or deploy the plan across the health continuum?

Answers to these questions can assist in determining if the team is headed in the right direction or whether it needs to revamp its course and focus. The novice CNL is most likely to lead or be a member of a unit-based or service group. Knowledge of how the organization uses teams to advance its mission, values, and goals is necessary.

Coalition or team building requires effective communication and interpersonal skills and knowledge of group dynamics. Successful groups will be judged by outcomes and their impact on organizational efficiency, effectiveness, customer satisfaction, and cost saving.

Group Dynamics

Group dynamics is the interactive behaviors of individuals within the context of a group. Like other important interpersonal relations, group dynamics involve individuals and the group as a whole. Group cohesiveness evolves over time and based on various issues previously discussed. Group dynamics extends beyond people meeting and agreeing or disagreeing to come to consensus about the purpose of the team, goal and outcome identification, timelines, and membership.

Empirical data of group development reveals an array of theories about group processes. Growing evidence also indicates that the survival of groups is based on a natural process in which they go through various phases or stages. For example, most people want to know something about team members, form some degree of interdependence to achieve team and personal goals, and effectively manage conflict.

The most frequently cited model of the developmental process is that of Bruce W. Tuckman (1965). Tuckman's model and group stages are as follows:

Forming: This is the orientation stage, in which members define interpersonal boundaries and task behaviors.

Storming: Resistance to group influence and task requirements occurs and is characterized by interpersonal conflicts.

Norming: Resistance abates, and group cohesiveness occurs; new expectations emerge, and new roles are accepted. Members feel free and comfortable sharing personal opinions, thoughts, and ideas.

Performing: Members become productive and work for the common good of the group. Interpersonal relations drive activities and results (Tuckman, 1965).

Adjourning: This dissolution stage refers to termination of roles and the completion of tasks. The group has successful attained its goals (Tuckman & Jensen, 1977).

This synopsis of Tuckman's (1965) model is helpful in understanding the normalcy of group dynamics and moving the team from the honeymoon period (forming); the storming, norming, and performing stages, in which the group cohesiveness and outcomes emerge, respectively; and the adjourning stage, in which the group terminates after it completes it purpose.

Developmental stages within organizations and interdisciplinary care coordination teams are useful in advancing the mission of the organization and health care. Group or team decision making involving tasks and strategies can be addressed by health promotion planning, education, policy development, and organizational support.

Conflict Management

Conflict occurs when two or more values, beliefs, or opinions are incongruous and reconciliation of differences has not occurred. Conflict frequently arises from stressful and emotional encounters or situations associated with diverse causes, such as those involving culture, gender, religion, age, health practices, health, socioeconomic issues, or education. Regardless of the cause, conflicts are a natural part of all relationships. Furthermore, they are necessary for health, personal development, and organizational growth. Resistance to change in healthcare systems is often led by individuals who are satisfied with the status quo and are threatened by change, new ideas, and other people. Societal and demographic changes increase the propensity of conflicts and opportunities to learn about others.

Predictably, unresolved conflict reduces productivity, is costly, lowers morale and self-esteem, increases apathy, and often results in inappropriate responses or even violence. Avoidance of conflict management often arises from passive behaviors, ineffective communication skills, apathy, or pretending it does not exist or is not worth resolving (see Table 6-2).

Management of Healthcare Environments

The final discussion centers on the management of healthcare environments through delegation, supervision, and interdisciplinary coordination of care. Management of care has been discussed extensively in previous sections of this chapter that covered leadership skills, effective communication, professional values, group dynamics, and conflict management. Specific issues that impact the new CNL within the organization vary and depend on educational preparation, clinical expertise, and leadership skills.

Organizational management requires looking at the "big picture" and intricacies that evolve from within and outside the healthcare system. Astute CNLs also develop alliances at the unit and leadership levels to glean knowledge about basic, standard operations and expectations within the role. For example, CNLs who choose to work primarily as administrators must have expert clinical skills to understand daily issues of taking care of patients and working with interdisciplinary teams. In the case of CNLs with an advanced practice background in mental health, the clinical and administrative components of their role are likely to help them form effective relationships and to lead interdisciplinary groups at the unit level, specialty unit level, and within the organization.

A CNL who is an advanced practice nurse with a critical care background can also integrate these competencies and work with staff at all levels within the organization. For instance, suppose that the new critical care nurse, John, who has difficulty managing his time and completing assignments in a timely manner, has been placed on a performance improvement plan. Laura, the CNL, can use her expertise in critical care nursing and administration to work with the John to discern areas of improvement while giving him assignments as a team member to explore ways of enhancing his time management and clinical skills to meet the terms of the performance improvement plan. Administratively, the CNL can also work with the nurse manager to help identify John's strengths and ways to strengthen his leadership skills to ensure a proactive response to staff members that are not performing as expected.

Frequently, the integration of clinical and administrative responsibilities requires the CNL to supervise others (as mentioned in the previous example), delegate responsibilities and duties, and facilitate interdisciplinary care coordination. *Delegation*, widely used in nursing, refers to the assignment of authority and responsibility to another person, usually a peer or subordinate, to perform specific activities. The individual who delegates is still accountable and responsible for the outcome of the delegated assignment. The decision to delegate infers that the person assigned to a specific task is competent to carry it out. If it's a technical assignment, such as performing a procedure, the CNL must observe and deem the individual competent to perform the assignment in his or her absence. Competence to perform delegated assignments is also the responsibility of the individual who agrees to the delegation. For instance, if the CNL is responsible for reporting critical lab values or performing waived tests, it is critical for the designated individual to demonstrate performance ability through verbal communication, written records, and observation. The same principles apply to delegated administrative assignments.

Interdisciplinary team coordination has been threaded throughout this chapter with various discussions about team building, leadership skills, and communications. As the CNL moves from novice to expert, communication and essential qualities remain the building blocks for team building, positive outcomes, and meeting the needs of internal and external consumers across the healthcare continuum.

Summary

- Regardless of role or practice setting, the CNL has an opportunity to establish alliances with individuals and consumers across the healthcare continuum.

- Effective communication will unlock many doors and facilitate organizational trust.
- Communication is a complex and interactive process.
- Leaders motivate others and generate change.
- Essential qualities are the foundation of nursing.
- Active listening is a critical communication tool.
- Assertiveness is an art that requires practice and fine tuning.
- Assertive communication is mutually respective and helps the CNL meet personal needs without disrespecting the rights of others.
- Professional values direct the manner in which we treat others, respect ourselves, and guide our practice and decision making.
- Leadership skills provide vast opportunities to deploy the CNL role across the healthcare continuum.
- Team building has demonstrated success and cost-effectiveness in advancing the needs of internal and external consumers and organization.

Reflection Questions

1. What does the organization expect regarding health care, internal and external consumers, quality, and safety?
2. Are providers expected to develop and implement evidence-based interventions and clinical outcomes?
3. What healthcare models are in place to address and manage complex patient problems and ensure appropriate monitoring, tracking, and trending quality improvement activities?
4. Does the organization embrace evidence-based practice? If not, why? By answering these questions, the CNL can generate ideas and develop a niche within the organization that is consistent with its mission, values, and expectations.
5. How can this knowledge guide the CNL to lead an initiative that facilitates implementation of evidence-based practice?
6. How can leadership skills be used to initiate this practice on one unit, additional units, and ultimately the entire organization?

Learning Activities

1. Select a mentor with strong leadership skills and shadow him or her during administrative or interdisciplinary group meetings.
2. Observe group dynamics in an interdisciplinary care coordination team to determine its developmental stage based on Tuckman's model.
3. Attend a new employee orientation session with senior leadership, and listen to their discussion about organization mission, values, and expectations from staff.
4. Shadow an advanced practice nurse in a leadership role, such as consultative liaison, and observe for active communication skills between patient, family, and staff.
5. Visit a community-based clinic, and shadow the administrative officer to learn how the clinic monitors and tracks quality indicators. Inquire about patient satisfaction scores (review trends and action plan to address low satisfaction scores).

References

Antai-Otong, D. (1997). Team building in a health care setting. *American Journal of Nursing, 97*(7), 48–51.

Antai-Otong, D. (2008). Therapeutic communication. In *Psychiatric nursing: Biological and behavioral concepts* (pp. 149–175). Clifton Park, NY: Delmar Thomson Learning.

Attaran, M., & Nguyen, T. T. (1999, July 1). Succeeding with self-managed work teams. *Industrial Management, 41*(4), 24–28.

Barker, A. M. (1992). *Transformational nursing leadership.* New York: National League for Nursing Press.

Biddle, B. J. (1986). Recent developments in role theory. *Annual Review of Sociology, 12,* 67–92.

Brown, C. E., Wickline, M. A., Ecoff, L., & Glaser, D. (2009). Nursing practice, knowledge, attitudes, and perceived barriers of evidence-based practice at an academic medical center. *Journal of Advanced Nursing, 65*(2), 371–381.

Chummun, H., & Tiran, D. (2008). Increasing research evidence in practice: A possible role for the consultant nurse. *Journal of Nursing Management, 16*(3), 327–333.

Cummings, G. G., Estabrooks, C. A., Midodzi, W. K., Wallin, L., & Hayduk, L. (2007). Influence of organizational characteristics and context on research utilization. *Nursing Research, 56*(Suppl. 4), S24–S39.

Engström, A., & Söderberg, S. (2007). Close relatives in intensive care from the perspective of critical care nurses. *Journal of Clinical Nursing, 16*(9), 1651–1659.

Kajermo, K. N., Undén, M., Gardulf, A., Eriksson, L. E., Orton, M. L., Arnetz, B. B., et al. (2008). Predictors of nurses' perceptions of barriers to research utilization. *Journal of Nursing Management, 16*(3), 305–314.

Koehn, M. L., & Lehman, K. (2008). Nurses' perceptions of evidence-based nursing practice. *Journal of Advanced Nursing, 62*(2), 209–215.

Krimsky, W. S., Mroz, I. B., McIlwaine, J. K., Surgenor, S. D., Christian, D., Corwin, H. L., et al. (2009). A model for increasing patient safety in the intensive care unit: Increasing the implementation rates of proven safety measures. *Quality and Safety in Health Care, 18*(1), 74–80.

Lloyd, J., Wise, M., Weeramanthri, T., & Nugus, P. (2009). The influence of professional values on the implementation of Aboriginal health policy. *Journal of Health Services Research & Policy, 14*(1), 6–12.

Maxwell, J. C. (1999). *The 21 indispensable qualities of a leader.* Nashville, TN: Thomas Nelson.

McIntosh, J., & Tolson, D. (2009). Leadership as part of the nurse consultant role: Banging the drum for patient care. *Journal of Clinical Nursing, 18*(2), 219–227.

Meltzer, L. J., Steinmiller, E., Simms, S., Grossman, M., Complex Care Consultation Team, & Li, Y. (2009). Staff engagement during complex pediatric medical care: The role of the patient, family, and treatment variables. *Patient Education Consultants, 74*(1), 77–83. Accessed at http://www.ncbi.nlm.nih.gov/pubmed/19209401

O'Connell, E., & Landers, M. (2008). The importance of critical care nurses' caring behaviours as perceived by nurses and relatives. *Intensive Critical Care Nursing, 24*(6), 349–358.

Scheetz, M. H., Bolon, M. K., Postelnick, M., Noskin, G. A., & Lee, T. A. (2009). Cost-effectiveness analysis of an antimicrobial stewardship team on bloodstream infections: A probabilistic analysis. *Journal of Antimicrobial Chemotherapy, 63*(4), 816–825. Accessed at http://jac.oxfordjournals.org/cgi/content/abstract/63/4/816

Tuckman, B. W. (1965). Developmental sequence in small groups. *Psychological Bulletin, 63*(6), 384–399.

Tuckman, B. W., & Jensen, M. A. C. (1977). Stages of small group development revisited. *Group and Organizational Studies*, 2(4), 419–427.

Watkins, M. (2003). *The first 90 days: Critical success strategies for new leaders at all levels.* Boston: Harvard Business School Press. Accessed at http://harvardbusinessonline.hbsp.harvard.edu/b01/en/common/item_detail.jhtml;jsessionid=DFTSHT4U01RDGAKRGWCB5VQBKE0YOISW?id=1105&_requestid=53590

Watson, J. (1988). *Human science and human care: A theory of nursing.* New York: National League of Nursing.

Yalom, I. D., & and Leszcz, M. (2005). *The theory and practice of group psychotherapy* (5th ed.). New York: Basic Books.

SEVEN

Quality Care and Risk Management

■ Patricia L. Thomas

■ **Learning Objectives**

■ Demonstrate an understanding of the CNL's role in microsystem quality improvement.

■ Gain confidence in assessing the microsystem, gathering tools, and collecting information necessary to implement systematic quality improvement efforts.

■ Establish the linkage between organizational goal, strategies, measurement, and communication of CNL efforts toward quality improvement.

■ Articulate the CNL's role in achieving a culture of safety and efficiency through process and quality improvement.

■ Evaluate quality improvement strategies in the CNL clinical immersion experience.

> "There is nothing so useless as doing efficiently that which should not be done at all."
>
> Peter Drucker

> "If you cannot describe what you are doing as a process, you do not know what you are doing."
>
> W. Edwards Deming

Key Terms

Quality improvement

Planning

Quality patient care and safety

Cyclical review

Needs assessment

Metrics and measurement evidence-
based practice

Microsystems

CNL Roles

Outcomes manager

Team manager

Systems analyst/risk anticipator

Coordinator of care

Information manager

Member of a profession

CNL Professional Values

Accountability

Outcome measurement

Quality improvement

Interdisciplinary teams

Integrity

Fiscal stewardship

Microsystem management

Evidence-based practice

Quality patient care and safety

Social justice

CNL Core Competencies

Healthcare systems and policy
designer/manager/coordinator
of care

Member of a profession

Critical thinking

Ethics

Assessment environment of care manager

Communication

Team leader

Information and healthcare technologies

Nursing technology and resource
management

Introduction

The American Association of Colleges of Nursing (AACN) introduced the role expectations of CNL with emphasis placed on the need to redesign the care delivery model for improved patient safety, effectiveness, and efficiency (2007). Inherent in the care delivery redesign process are multidisciplinary team members committed to excellence and quality improvement quantified through metrics and measurement. By acknowledging the need to decrease fragmentation of care in the delivery system, processes underlying care delays, redundancy, or gaps in service, and dissatisfaction within provider, patients, and stakeholders groups, quality improvement offers a framework and methods to support changes in interrelated systems aimed toward better clinical and financial outcomes.

Several landmark studies have influenced the trends in quality improvement to address real and pressing concerns in the U.S. health system. In 1999 the Institute of Medicine (IOM) published *To Err Is Human: Building a Safer Health System*, which highlighted that between 44,000 and 98,000 Americans die each year as a result of medical errors—exceeding the loss of lives from car accidents, breast cancer, and AIDS (IOM, 1999). Additionally, the cost of preventable errors resulting in injury was between $17 billion and $29 billion. The fragmentation of the healthcare delivery system was identified as a major contributor to these errors. With these findings, the focus shifted to building a safer, outcomes-driven care delivery system relying on quality improvement tools to increase efficiency, cost-effectiveness, and high performance (AACN, 2007; The Joint Commission, 2008).

A second IOM report, *Crossing the Quality Chasm: A New Health System for the 21st Century*, made an urgent call for change that emphasized safety, effectiveness, patient-centeredness, and care that is timely, efficient, and equitable (IOM, 2001). This landmark study stressed the environment of care and systems issues as pivot points that negatively impacted safety and effectiveness, noting that the care patients receive in today's healthcare delivery system has become increasingly complex, with nurses simultaneously interacting with multiple systems, processes, and technologies (Nelson, Batalden, & Godfrey, 2007; Wiggins, 2008). In a follow-up report, *Health Professions Education: A Bridge to Quality*, the IOM recommended that health professionals be educated to deliver patient-centered care as members of an interdisciplinary team, emphasizing implementation of evidence-based practices, quality improvement practices, and informatics (AACN, 2007).

In 2008, The Joint Commission published a report, *Health Care at the Crossroads: Guiding Principles for the Development of the Hospital of the Future*, emphasizing the increasing complexity of care delivery and the pace of change and innovations that make it difficult for clinicians to keep pace. Recognizing that hospitalized patients have higher acuity, greater comorbid conditions in need of management, and shortened hospital stays, The Joint Commission highlighted that the average length of stay decreased 25% since the 1980s. At the same time, the Food and Drug Administration approved more than 500,000 new medical devices. Advances in pharmaceuticals and genomic developments have exploded into the health delivery landscape during this time period as well. Although advances in technology help improve patient outcomes, the volume of technologies and the requisite knowledge to manage them have made care delivery more complex, with sometimes unforeseen opportunities for error. This multifaceted complexity weighs heavily on conscientious clinicians. To respond to these demands, The Joint Commission identified the CNL as the clinician suited to manage the "real-time" care of patients within the microsystem to ensure evidence-based practices and quality improvement principles, measurement, and evaluation to improve patient care outcomes.

The CNL role creates an opportunity for new care models and team configurations in every delivery setting. Regulatory and accreditation pressures to increase safety and reduce costs are mounting as we examine health outcomes. Unprecedented attention to cost, dwindling human and financial resources, and acknowledgment of increasing complexity underpin the desire to systematically address historical practices that present threats to patient safety (The Joint Commission, 2008; Newhouse, 2006; Rusch & Bakewell-Sachs, 2007). The assumptions underpinning the CNL role competencies are translated into daily operational performance at the point of care. Cost evaluation, return on investment, and cost/benefit analyses will be essential to validate the CNL impact on cost reductions in an environment in which pay for performance and the expectation of reducing errors, and improving safety and efficiency are paramount to future organizational success (Haase-Herrick, 2005; Hwang & Herndon, 2007).

Background

The AACN, in collaboration with nurse executives, health systems, and educators, proposed the CNL as nursing solution to address gaps in healthcare quality by addressing patient needs, safety, and quality improvement through a systematic and deliberate approach to implementing evidence-based practice, quality management, and clinical leadership at the point of care. CNLs are prepared as advanced generalists accountable for identifying outcomes of practice on their units. This can be accomplished by participating in a range of quality improvement projects aimed to collect and create evidence, lead multidisciplinary teams, and incorporate interventions with the greatest likelihood to produce high-quality care outcomes (AACN, 2007; Bowcutt, Wall, & Goolsby, 2006).

Supporting a Culture of Safety

With general agreement that patient safety needs improvement, it is important for healthcare providers to have a consistent, clear, and concise definition of quality. Lohr (1990) defined *quality* as "the degree to which health services for individuals and populations increase the likelihood of desired health outcomes and are consistent with current professional knowledge" (p. 4). Systematic, deliberate, and defined methods will be needed to measure, understand, improve, and communicate internal progress at the unit and organization levels. Regulatory agencies and groups external to the organization, including professional organizations, payers, and policy makers, will also need this information to make policy decisions based on clear measurements, shared goals, and systematic approaches toward improvement (Hwang & Herndon, 2007; Newhouse, 2006).

CNLs are positioned to mentor, coach, and guide multidisciplinary teams to enact the paradigm shift necessary to sustain a culture of safety found in the application of evidence-based practices and quality improvement. In addition to advanced clinical knowledge, CNLs examine the care delivery system from the perspective of individual patients or a microsystem population framework recognizing the interrelated functions of process, information management, and outcomes (AACN, 2007; Nelson et al., 2007).

Distinguishing Quality Improvement, Evidence-Based Practice, and the CNL Role

Quality improvement is known by many names but holds in common the real-life experiences and data within the context of an organization to rapidly cycle through a defined process to evaluate outcomes that are actionable (McLaughlin & Kaluzny, 2006; Newhouse, 2007). The terms *continuous quality improvement, total quality management, performance improvement,* and *process improvement* are often used interchangeably to describe efforts geared toward data-driven, process-oriented, outcome-focused activities. These efforts were originally established in the business world and have recently been applied in the healthcare industry. Oftentimes, quality improvement is offered as a framework to examine long-standing clinical and systems issues in a different way (McLaughlin & Kaluzny, 2006; Nelson et al., 2007).

The key feature of quality improvement is the cyclical nature of the process designed to evaluate workflow and processes built from value-added actions performed by work teams in a system (Hedges, 2006; McLaughlin & Kaluzny, 2006; Newhouse, 2007). Quality improvement processes do not meet the standards or rigor found in scientific research and have neither theoretical underpinnings nor an aim to generate new knowledge. Rather, quality improvement aims to bring individuals that work together into a venue in which systematic review and evaluation of work processes can be examined in a cyclical fashion as a means to evaluate and improve established practices and outcomes (Hedges, 2006; Newhouse, 2007).

Philosophical Elements of Quality Improvement

Continuous quality improvement holds several characteristics that are evident in organizations (McLaughlin and Kaluzny, 2006):

- Strategic focus drawing on the mission and values of the organization;
- A customer focus directed toward patients, providers, and stakeholders;
- A systems perspective, revealing emphasis on the interdependence of interacting processes that influence outcomes;
- Data driven analysis emphasizing the gathering of objective data to influence decision making;
- Team involvement inclusive of representatives who implement current work processes and those who will implement the resulting workflow change;
- Multiple causations requiring identification of root causes;
- Sets of solutions identified to enhance system functions and outcomes;
- Process optimization supported by alignment of tools and structures to evaluate interventions;
- Continuous improvement supported by ongoing analysis of outcomes directed toward ongoing modification of processes to enhance system performance; and
- Organizational learning so the capacity to generate future improvements is enhanced.

Several quality improvement methodologies reside in health systems, identified as *Lean*, *Six Sigma*, or *Total Quality Management* structures. Irrespective of the quality improvement methodology selected by an organization, there are eight common steps in quality improvement (McLaughlin & Kaluzny, 2006; Newhouse, 2006):

1. Establishing a clear and defined aim or purpose;
2. Reviewing the literature;
3. Examining current resources to facilitate quality improvement;
4. Mapping the current processes;
5. Analyzing the root cause;
6. Selecting appropriate tools for process analysis;
7. Selecting measures and metrics (baseline and outcome); and
8. Conducting a rapid cyclical review of the plan, data, interventions, and outcomes.

Defined Aim or Purpose

Although a clear purpose or aim in any project seems logical, this is a part of quality improvement that can lead to frustration when project teams engage in work. Because the team is comprised of individuals from varied disciplines, many assumptions underlie how we define and view clinical issues. Additionally, because processes are complex and interrelated, it is easy for a team to lose focus or expand the project scope if the aim or purpose is not clearly and explicitly defined.

When creating an aim or purpose for a quality improvement team, answering *who*, *what*, *when*, *where*, and *how* is key. *Who* refers to those affected by the concern; *what* refers to the problem identified; *when* refers to when the issue occurs; *where* refers to the specific unit or location of the concern; and *how* refers to the measures, metrics, or standards that let you know you have an issue. Once the team can establish these parameters, elevator discussions, or concise yet informative language suitable to a conversation that lasts the duration of an elevator ride, can be crafted. Additionally, when the team starts to drift into processes or topics that do not relate specifically and directly to the purpose or aim of the team, issues for the "parking lot" can be documented for future discussion or communication to other project teams.

Review of the Literature

Newhouse (2007) defined evidence-based practice (EBP) as a problem-solving approach to clinical decision making that integrates the best available scientific evidence with the best available experiential evidence from patients and practitioners, incorporating the organization's culture, internal and external influences on practice, and critical thinking that supports judicious application of the evidence to the care of an individual, a population of patients, or the system. EBP and research inform quality improvement through review of the literature. By providing interventions with great likelihood of success, both research and evidence-based practices inform quality improvement (Newhouse, 2007).

Central to the CNL role is the expectation that clinical practice and interventions be evidence-based. Driven from past experiences in failing to achieve consistent and sustainable improvements, and increasing regulatory demands to demonstrate the inclusion of evidence in processes, protocols, and policies, evidence-based practices are gaining attention. National patient safety goals, based in Joint Commission requirements and supported by the National Quality Forum, set the overarching goal for establishing EBP as the norm in clinical care (CMMS, 2009; The Joint Commission, 2008).

Examination of Resources to Facilitate Improvement

When undertaking a quality improvement initiative, it is important to explore, examine, and establish both internal and external resources to support any project. Internal resources can include individuals from quality management departments, finance, information services, the library, and the education department. Books, Internet sites, and discussions with members of the interdisciplinary team who have had experience with quality improvement activities can provide important contacts to support a team's efforts. External resources include professional organizations, Internet resources, quality improvement organizations, and members of other industries with knowledge in quality management or root cause analysis.

Mapping of Current Processes

Several methods for mapping current processes exist. When initiating the mapping process, CNLs will engage members of the interdisciplinary team in exercises to identify, define, and document process steps, decision points, and inputs from other departments or disciplines that lead to the current outcomes (McLaughlin & Kaluzny, 2006). This stage involves a detail-specific discussion among members of the team to capture the complexity of the process intended for improvement.

Root Cause Analysis

The Joint Commission established expectations for organizations to proactively identify high-risk processes likely to contribute to errors. Within this process is the realization that systems and processes contribute to adverse events and errors. Because quality improvement initiatives are focused on addressing processes, it is important to use systematic approaches to guide teams in identifying the root cause or process that breaks down and leads to an undesired result. Once a process flow is completed, further analysis of each process is required to identify the underlying cause or step in a process that sets into motion a cause and effect that drives an occurrence or problem. Drilling down on process steps to identify a root cause can be accomplished using different tools, but cause and effect or fishbone diagrams are most common. Fishbone diagrams delineate the causes of a situation centered on predefined categories of people, materials, methods, machinery, and policy (McLaughlin & Kaluzny, 2006; Shaw, Elliott, Isaacson, & Murphy, 2003).

Selection of Appropriate Tools

There are several tools used to represent data collected before, during, and after quality improvement efforts are undertaken. Each tool has a distinct purpose and provides a fact-based approach to identify concerns, propose solutions, and monitor outcomes of the process changes. The most common tools are include brainstorming, cause-and-effect diagrams, Pareto charts, control charts, process flow diagrams, fishbone diagrams, surveys, pie charts, histograms, and run charts (McLaughlin & Kaluzny, 2006; Newhouse, 2007; Shaw et al., 2003).

Selection of Measures and Metrics

Measurement and metrics are the foundation to quality improvement because they are the basis for evaluating the impact of quality improvement activities. Defining the metrics at baseline is the starting point for quality activities because these measures typically inform and define how a problem was recognized. Equally important are the primary and secondary metrics the quality improvement team selects as they modify processes to achieve the team's goals and purpose. Metrics can include clinical indicators of care and process or business metrics (McLaughlin & Kaluzny, 2006; Nelson et al., 2007; Newhouse, 2006).

Technology, and therefore electronic medical records and informatics, have been infused into the care arena at a rapid pace during the last decade. Clinicians are often bombarded with more data than they could possibly analyze and review. With this in mind, it is important to CNLs to consider how information is gathered, where it is stored, and what tools, methods, and resources are available to access data. When reviewing data stored in data warehouses, repositories, and databases, it is important to clarify terms and data definitions to ensure consistency and understanding of how data will be used in the quality improvement process (Bakken, Cimino, & Hripcsak, 2004).

Although nurses are generally comfortable assessing clinical outcomes and indicators of care, it is important for CNLs to incorporate business metrics and measurements when planning quality improvement projects. These measures are important to the administrators and regulators of care accustomed to quantifying and articulating value at a systems level (Haase-Herrick, 2005; Hwang & Herndon, 2007). Quantifying the return on investment and impacts on costs of care, and articulating system improvements could establish the value of the CNL role in organizations. With rising pressures regarding pay for performance, trended outcomes of care in public reporting, and rising interest from accreditation and consumer groups, selection of business indicators aimed at cost-effectiveness and efficiency are essential.

Rapid Cycle Review

A cornerstone and distinguishing characteristic of quality improvement, rapid cycle review encourages continuous and ongoing efforts to improve outcomes. The plan, do, check, act (PDCA) cycle is frequently referenced in quality improvement methodologies. Discussed by Deming (and attributed to Shewhart's work at Bell Laboratories), the PDCA cycle of improvement offers a cyclical process to structure tests of change identified by team members as being most likely to improve outcomes in a disciplined and rapid manner (McLaughlin & Kaluzny, 2006). The *plan* involves defining the problem, examining the processes that contribute to it, and devising a plan to address the problem. *Do* involves identifying the steps in a plan and carrying them out. *Check* involves analyzing the data collected to summarize what was learned. *Act* involves examining outcomes with an eye toward further modifications so that the cycle can be initiated again to refine and bring further improvements (McLaughlin & Kaluzny, 2006; Nelson et al., 2007).

Relevance of the Microsystem

Microsystems are defined as the smallest functional unit on the frontline of healthcare delivery systems. The clinical microsystem provides the direct care to patients and families, establishing the essential building blocks of the organization. It is within this microsystem that the quality of care is defined and the reputation of the organization is created (Nelson et al., 2006).

Microsystems include members of the interdisciplinary team in various roles who work together on a regular basis to provide care to discrete subpopulations of patients. Each microsystem has business and clinical aims, linked processes, and a shared information environment that produces performance outcomes (Nelson et al., 2006). Microsystems are represented in all practice settings and specialties and evolve over time but always have a patient at their center. Microsystems vary widely in terms of quality, safety, and costs because they are embedded in a context in which providers, support staff, information, and processes converge to support individuals who provide care to meet the unique and individual health needs of patients and families. Microsystems are loosely or tightly connected to one another and are the functional, interdependent systems that create an organization or macrosystem (Nelson et al., 2007).

As Tornabeni, Stanhope, and Wiggins (2008) noted, "The CNL role focuses on understanding the interdependency of all disciplines providing care and the need to tap into the expertise of the team, rather than individual providers" (p. 107). By understanding the roles of the interdisciplinary team, the CNL laterally integrates the team to provide patient-centered care. CNLs use their interpersonal communication skills, clinical leadership skills, and knowledge of group dynamics to facilitate care, leveraging their knowledge of internal and external resources to provide lateral integration.

Assessment of the Microsystem for Selection of Quality Improvement Projects

Many tools have been created to support CNLs in the assessment of their microsystems. Irrespective of the tool selected, a thorough and systematic assessment is needed before embarking on a quality improvement project. The microsystem assessment elements to be examined include the following: unit descriptors; skills, composition, and competence of team members; presence of formal and informal leaders; interdisciplinary team relationships and communication; accountability and control over practice; support for education; experience with quality improvement processes and resources; and readiness for change.

The 5-P (purpose, patients, professionals, processes, and patterns) framework offers a deliberate structure for clinicians to assess microsystems in a systematic manner. Each *P* has a definition associated with it, and these categories set a framework to inform the selection of improvement themes and aims. To be most effective, the exploration of the five *P*s should include all the members of a clinical microsystem. Nelson and colleagues (2007) offer a series of questions and exercises to lead interdisciplinary teams through the microsystem assessment to establish the condition of the microsystem (health), making obvious the areas requiring attention (diagnosis) and solutions (treatment) to be evaluated by the team (follow-up; p. 265).

Systematic and Purposeful Identification of Quality Improvement Initiatives

When considering the initiatives to improve quality and safety, project selection in an organization is of paramount importance. By using a gap analysis or microsystem assessment, CNLs can align quality improvement efforts in the microsystem to the strategic initiatives and organizational goals while focusing attention on the front lines to impact change. The CNL is in a unique position to manage change, apply quality improvement methods, and incorporate team learning by leading interdisciplinary members through a disciplined, systematic approach of problem identification, process analysis, measurement, and evaluation that is meaningful in daily operations.

A potential pitfall for CNLs is the identification of quality improvement projects that extend beyond the microsystem. Scoping a project through a defined aim or purpose at the onset of quality improvement activities is essential to success. Because there are many priorities that overlap at the organizational level, concentrating on improvements at the microsystem level is key. Problem identification through brainstorming with members of the microsystem team is a mechanism to support unit-level activities that will be meaningful and appropriate for CNL intervention (Rusch & Bakewell-Sachs, 2007; Thompson & Lulham, 2007).

Structure for Monitoring Quality Improvement Projects

Many organizations have quality departments that distribute quality reports monthly, quarterly, or annually as a part of a quality dashboard, benchmarking, or quality report card process. In addition to these contributions, many quality departments distribute reports for quality improvement initiatives and regulatory obligations. Because there is a wealth of knowledge contained in these departments, before engaging in a quality improvement project, the CNL team leader should explore the tools, report development, and distribution supports that might be available.

Team Leader Tools for Success

Once the philosophy of quality improvement has been embraced and the tenets of quality improvement have been articulated, the progress toward improvement needs to be monitored and evaluated. Irrespective of the methodology selected to guide the organizational quality improvements, team member roles, responsibilities, and ground rules need to be discussed and documented. This step is commonly avoided or driven by assumptions, but this is a critical mistake. If CNLs are going to embrace quality improvement, it is essential to set team expectations and responsibilities from the onset of the group's work. The documents created during this phase of the team's interactions will be referenced throughout the quality improvement process as the agreed-on guiding principles, rules, and accountabilities each team member holds.

Several forms or documents can be found to record the team's expectations. At a minimum, the team will want to identify the team leader, the secretary (responsible for documenting and distributing meeting minutes and agendas), and the responsibilities of each team member. Attendance requirements, frequency of meetings, length of meetings, and commitment to completing work between meetings are the focal points for discussion among the team members.

Team Charter

Searching the Internet for "team charters" provides a wealth of templates or formats for teams to consider if the organization does not have a preferred or approved template. A charter is a written agreement defining what your team is going to accomplish and how success will be measured. The charter focuses the team's efforts and documents the expectations that team members have for one another. By using the team charter, discussion between multidisciplinary team members can be guided to include key focal points in team dynamics and important issues can be agreed upon before the team engages in the quality improvement project. A signed charter indicates the formal beginning of a project and a commitment to one another.

Irrespective of the template used, the team charter includes the following information (Shaw et al., 2003):

- Project title
- Description of the project in terms the team understands
- A defined scope of the project and deliverables
- Problem to be addressed/business case
- Success criteria (defined goals and measurable outcomes anticipated)
- Time commitment (frequency of meetings, length of meetings, expected completion date)
- Team member roles (team leader, secretary, timekeeper, and sponsor/champion)
- Minute management process

- Decision-making process
- Conflict management process
- Communication plans (Who will get information and when?)
- Expectations of team members (review of minutes, checking e-mail/voice mail, response and turnaround times, preparation prior to meetings, completing assignments)

Team Agenda/Meeting Minutes Template

The team agenda should be created based on the goals of the team during each phase of the quality improvement project, and it should proactively identify time allotted to each activity on the agenda and the person responsible for leading the discussion. Once at the team meeting, the agenda template can be completed to reflect decisions made, and action steps or follow-up items. Here is a sample template:

Sample Agenda and Meeting Minutes Template

Team Project Name

Date, Time, and Location of Meeting

Attendees:

Agenda and Meeting Minutes

Team Project Name _____

Date _____ Time _____

Location of Meeting _____

Attendees _____

_____

Topic/ Presenter	Time Allowed	Discussion Points	Follow-Up/ Action Step	Due Date

Team Ground Rules

Although most professionals hold common beliefs about group process and goal attainment, ground rules provide the boundaries for how team members will interact. Many organizations have established ground rules for team interactions based on their mission and shared values. Although these ground rules provide basic tenets for group interactions, it is important to offer team members the ability to modify rules to reflect what the team members believe the guiding principles should be.

Common content for ground rules include the following (Shaw et al., 2003):

- Every person has a valuable viewpoint.
- Every person will make a unique contribution to the team.
- Team members will listen attentively when other team members speak.
- Team members will speak one at a time and not engage in sidebar discussions.
- Organizational titles and positions will not be recognized during the team meetings. All members of the team are of equal importance and influence.
- All team members will accept responsibility for assignments and due dates.
- All team members will be treated with respect.
- At the close of each meeting, the team will evaluate the team process.

CNLs are positioned to monitor the improvement activities from the team leader position as a coordinator and manager of care through teaching, guidance, mentoring, and leveraging the language of the improvement process. Effective use of team tools can set expectations and provide elements that document activities and progress that lead to the attainment of project goals.

Linking Quality Improvement to the Clinical Immersion Experience

Embedded in the CNL role are expectations of accountability for patient client-centered, cost-effective care across practice settings, and measurable outcomes that demonstrate improved safety, quality, and evidence-based practice. The CNL curriculum supports the development of clinical leaders who can manage change by leading members of the interdisciplinary team in complex care environments (AACN, 2007; Rusch & Bakewell-Sachs, 2007).

All CNLs are required to complete 400–500 clinical hours throughout their educational experience, with 300–400 hours devoted to a clinical immersion experience.

During the clinical immersion experience, the student enacts the CNL role and competencies in an organization (AACN, 2007; Rusch & Bakewell-Sachs, 2007). Although quality improvement may be offered as a separate course in the curriculum or threaded throughout the educational experience in several courses, the culmination of the CNL clinical immersion experience is grounded in principles demonstrated through quality improvement projects. As members of the nursing profession, CNLs will be expected to identify areas for improvement within the care delivery system, assess and plan meaningful change at the microsystem level, and measure clinical and financial outcomes to demonstrate improved outcomes that align with strategic organizational goals aimed at improvement in cost, quality, and safety.

As clinical leaders and members of the nursing profession, CNLs are also expected to participate in self-evaluation and reflective thinking (AACN, 2007). This would include examining individually held assumptions, values, and beliefs with an open mind, supported by the use of critical thinking skills to explore different perspectives, solutions, and options offered by members of the interdisciplinary team or the literature. The clinical immersion experience offers CNL students a venue to share the outcomes of quality improvement activities as well as the reflective practice, learning, and insights gained related to leading teams, evaluating practice and implementing evidence-based practices, and guiding or mentoring others in quality improvement processes aimed to address patient safety and improved care delivery. Documents assembled during the quality improvement process can then become a part of the students' clinical immersion portfolio.

Monitoring Tools for the CNL

Clinical logs and journals can be accessed to support the CNL in reflective practice during a quality course or as part of the clinical immersion experience. Documenting progress toward established goals in a deliberate and systematic fashion can provide valuable insights into the enactment and transition to the CNL role.

Clinical Logs

Clinical logs, completed on a weekly or biweekly basis, provide detail directed toward time management, clarity of purpose, and next steps as the CNL progresses through the quality improvement process. Below is a template offered to structure the content of the clinical log. The information in this log can be shared with CNL faculty or the quality improvement sponsor or champion.

Name _____

Additional lines can be added as needed.
Below is a template:

Date	Activities/Actions	Objective Number(s)	Time Spent (Hours/Minutes)

Name_____

Total Hours This Week _____

Cumulative Hours (Hours Completed to Date) _____

Description of Activities/Actions

Whom did you meet with?

What did you do?

What were the obstacles/barriers? What is needed to address them?

What are your goals for next week?

Reflective Journals

Journals are not time logs but rather a place for reflection, personal and professional awareness, and recording what has been learned during your clinical time. The reflective journal serves several purposes, including a place to record one's thoughts and reactions to course content, clinical applications, events, professional activities, and insights. According to Lasater and Nielson (2009), guided reflective journals offer professional nurses a way to view situations from multiple perspectives, search for alternative explanations of events, and use evidence to support or evaluate a decision or position.

Reflective journaling requires thought and introspection on the part of the CNL. A reflective journal is not a diary, resource book, or log of daily activities. It is a place to record experiences, ideas, and insights to allow an introspective view of the team dynamics, clinical leader responsibilities, and progress toward goals. A journal chronicles self-assessment, self-evaluation, and evolving perspective. The following list offers a starting point for reflective journaling content:

- Explore questions for inquiry that are important to you.
- Record significant experiences, including associated feelings and thoughts.
- Analyze patterns and relationships.
- Appreciate learning and celebrate success.
- Respond to new ideas.
- Examine your assumptions, beliefs, and values.
- Consider alternative perspectives.
- Develop personal theories.
- Take thoughtful action.

Thoughtful reflection is an ongoing process. Your journal is not a showpiece. Like your learning, it will always be a work in progress. Approach it with curiosity and openness.

Conclusion

With increasing national demands from regulators, payers, and consumers to support effectiveness of interventions to improve patient safety and quality of care, change efforts formed by quality improvement initiatives provide a systematic, disciplined, and reliable process to support decision making and measurement aimed to improve patient care quality in the healthcare delivery system. Developing a data-driven, outcomes-oriented structure grounded in role accountability will be essential. CNLs are well positioned to lead multidisciplinary teams in their efforts to implement quality improvement at the microsystem level.

Summary

- As coordinators of care with a system of care focus, CNLs have responsibility to lead interdisciplinary teams in quality improvement initiatives.
- Irrespective of the quality methods employed in an organization, quality improvement relies on a systematic and disciplined approach to understanding care processes.
- Evidence-based practices inform the selection of appropriate interventions and inform quality improvement to support quality care and data-driven outcomes.

Reflection Questions

1. What part of the quality improvement process do you feel most prepared for? What part do you feel least prepared for?
2. What resources are available in your organization to assist you with quality improvement?
3. How do you see the CNL interacting with other members of the clinical team to advance quality improvement and evidence-based practices?

Learning Activities

1. Interview a member of your organization's quality improvement department. Identify the quality methods, tools, and measurement techniques used in the organization.
2. Locate the quality reports and metrics that are distributed to leaders throughout the organization. Identify three metrics that you believe the CNL could impact.
3. Outline the steps you would undertake if you were going to develop a quality improvement plan to address a metric CNLs could address.

Recommended Reading

Hughes, R. G. (n.d.). Tools and strategies for quality improvement and patient safety. In *Patient safety and quality: An evidence-based handbook for nurses*. Available at http://www.ahrq.gov/qual/nurseshdbk/docs/HughesR_QMBMP.pdf

Web Sites That Address Quality and Safety

- http://www.ahrq.gov (Agency for Healthcare Quality and Research); see also http://www.ahrq.gov/qual; and http://www.ahrq.gov/qual/toolkit
- http://www.cms.hhs.gov (Centers for Medicare & Medicaid Services)
- http://dms.dartmouth.edu/cms (Dartmouth Institute for Health Policy and Clinical Practice); see also http://dms.dartmouth.edu/cms/toolkits; and http://dms.dartmouth.edu/cms/materials/workbooks/action_guide
- http://ihi.org (Institute for Healthcare Improvement); see also http://ihi.org/IHI/Topics/Improvement/ImprovementMethods/HowToImprove; http://ihi.org/IHI/Topics/Improvement/ImprovementMethods/Measures; and http://ihi.org/IHI/Topics/Improvement/ImprovementMethods/Tools

- http://www.jointcommission.org (The Joint Commission)
- http://www.qualityforum.org (National Quality Forum)

References

American Association of Colleges of Nursing (AACN). (2007, February). *White paper on the education and role of the clinical nurse leader.* Retrieved March 20, 2009, from http://www.aacn.nche.edu/Publications/WhitePapers/CNL2-07.pdf

Bakken, S., Cimino, J., & Hripcsak, G. (2004). Promoting patient safety and enabling evidence-based practice through informatics. *Medical Care, 42*(Suppl. 2), II-49–II-56.

Bowcutt, M., Wall, J., & Goolsby, M. (2006). The clinical nurse leader: Promoting patient-centered outcomes. *Nursing Administration Quarterly, 30*(2), 156–161.

Centers for Medicare & Medicaid Services (CMS). (2009). *Medicaid and CHIP quality practices: General information.* Retrieved March 27, 2009, from http://www.cms.hhs.gov/Medicaid SCHIPQualPrac/03_evidencebasedcare.asp

Haase-Herrick, K. (2005). The opportunities of stewardship. *Nursing Administration Quarterly, 29*(2), 115–118.

Hedges, C. (2006). Research, evidence-based practice, and quality improvement: The 3-legged stool. *AACN Advanced Critical Care, 17*(4), 457–459.

Hwang, R., & Herndon, J. (2007). The business case for patient safety. *Clinical Orthopaedics and Related Research, 457,* 21–34.

Institute of Medicine (IOM). (1999). *To err is human: Building a safer health system.* Washington, DC: National Academies Press.

Institute of Medicine (IOM). (2001). *Crossing the quality chasm: A new health system for the 21st century.* Washington, DC: National Academies Press.

The Joint Commission. (2008). *Health care at the crossroads: Guiding principles for the development of the hospital of the future.* Retrieved February 25, 2009, from http://www.jointcom mission.org/NR/rdonlyres/1C9A7079-7A29-4658-B80D-A7DF8771309B/0/Hosptal_ Future.pdf

Lasater, K., & Nielson, A. (2009). Reflective journaling for clinical judgment development and evaluation. *Journal of Nursing Education, 48*(1), 40–44.

Lohr, K. (1990). *Medicare: A strategy for quality assurance.* Washington, DC: National Academies Press.

McLaughlin, C. P., & Kaluzny, A. D. (2006). *Continuous quality improvement in health care: Theory, implementations, and applications* (3rd ed.). Sudbury, MA: Jones and Bartlett.

Nelson, E., Batalden, P., & Godfrey, M. (2007). *Quality by design: A clinical microsystems approach.* San Francisco: Jossey-Bass.

Newhouse, R. (2006). Selecting measures for safety and quality improvement initiatives. *Journal of Nursing Administration, 36*(3), 109–113.

Newhouse, R. (2007). Diffusing confusion among evidence-based practice, quality improvement, and research. *Journal of Nursing Administration, 37*(10), 432–435.

Rusch, L., & Bakewell-Sachs, S. (2007). The CNL: A gateway to better care. *Nursing Management, 38*(4), 32, 34, 36–37.

Shaw, P., Elliott, C., Isaacson, P., & Murphy, E. (2003). *Quality and performance improvement in healthcare: A tool for programmed learning* (2nd ed.). Chicago: American Health Information Management Association.

Thompson, P., & Lulham, K. (2007). Clinical nurse leader and clinical nurse specialist role delineation in the acute care setting. *Journal of Nursing Administration, 37*(10), 429–431.

Tornabeni, J., Stanhope, M., & Wiggins, M. (2008). The CNL vision. *Journal of Nursing Administration, 36*(3), 103–108.

Wiggins, M. S. (2008). The partnership care delivery model: An examination of the core concept and the need for a new model of care. *Journal of Nursing Management, 16*(5), 629–638.

EIGHT

Using Evidence to Guide Clinical Nurse Leader Practice

■ Carol Boswell and Sharon Cannon

■ **Learning Objectives**

■ Discuss decision-making theories within the clinical area.

■ Analyze key evidence-based practice concepts as they apply to the CNL role.

■ Utilize outcome evaluation strategies for the provision of patient care.

> "Most people spend more time and energy going around problems than in trying to solve them."
>
> Henry Ford

Key Terms

Decision making theories

Evidence-based practice

Research

Analysis

SWOT

Intuition

Political model

Bureaucratic model

Normative/prescriptive theory

Satisficing theory

Evidence

Outcomes

Intuition

Problem solving

PICOT

Rational model

Collegial model

Garbage can model

Descriptive/behavioral theory

Optimizing theory

CNL Roles

Clinician

Client advocate

Information manager

Team manager

Lifelong learner

Outcome manager

Educator

Systems analysis/risk anticipator

Member of a profession

CNL Professional Values

Altruism

Human dignity

Accountability

Integrity

CNL Core Competencies

Critical thinking

Illness and disease management

Ethics

Healthcare systems and policy

Communication

Information and healthcare technologies

Human diversity

Provider and manager of care

Designer/manager/coordinator of care Member of a profession

Nursing technology and resource management

Introduction

According to the American Association of Colleges of Nursing (AACN; 2007), "the CNL is a leader in the health care delivery system across all settings in which health care is delivered, not just the acute care setting" (p. 6). The AACN endeavored to clarify the mission of the CNL by creating assumptions for functionality of the role. As the AACN established the assumptions, evidence-based practice is threaded throughout the following assumptions:

Assumption 2: Client care outcomes are the measure of quality practice.

Assumption 3: Practice guidelines are based on evidence.

Assumption 5: Information will maximize self-care and client decision making.

Assumption 6: Nursing assessment is the basis for theory and knowledge development.

Assumption 10: The CNL must assume guardianship for the nursing profession.

The CNL has the responsibility and expectation to make a difference not only in the acute care setting but across the healthcare delivery spectrum. Each setting in which nursing leaders are engaged in the delivery of health care to individuals, families, or community, the obligation to incorporate sound and tested health practices is essential. Assumption 10 places an important obligation for the CNL to protect and preserve the art and science of nursing. As a professional, the CNL must elevate the distinction and magnitude of the provision of nursing care to the level of evidence-based practice. Oman, Duran, and Fink (2008) stated that "evidence-based practice has become the cornerstone of nursing practice worldwide" (p. 47). No longer can the nursing profession depend on "that's how we have always done it" as a reason for providing substandard health care to the public. Every skill and task undertaken within the realm of nursing should be supported by evidence.

AACN (2007) has challenged nursing educators and professionals to accept the "unparalleled opportunity and capability to address the critical issues that face the nation's current health care system" (p. 3). Only by accepting the challenge to transform nursing care, established on facts and evidence, can the profession have an impact on changing healthcare delivery methods. Because the CNL is envisioned as functioning within the microsystem, these individuals have the explicit picture of the challenges and opportunities evident at the bedside and within the work environment. Schoenfelder (2007) stated that "delivering nursing care and services that are based on the best current evidence is characteristic of clinical leadership" (p. 11). The individuals practicing at the unit level have to be encouraged to participate in these critical healthcare discussions concerning the future provision of health and nursing care.

Although many definitions for evidence-based practice are currently available, each of the definitions has key aspects as foundational. These key aspects are as follows: a decision-making process is employed, a clinical focus is understood, evidence is the foundation, and client involvement is imperative (Boswell & Cannon, 2007). Each of these aspects is clearly denoted within the assumptions established for the CNL:

- research/evidence—Assumption 3,
- clinical expertise—Assumption 10, and
- client preferences—Assumption 5.

With the changing face of health care resulting in the need to discover and implement new strategies, the nursing profession, led by the CNL, should be instrumental in evaluating and implementing appropriate and effective modifications into the provision of nursing science. The CNL must assume the "accountability for healthcare outcomes for a specific group of clients within a unit or setting through the assimilation and application of research-based information to design, implement, and evaluate client plans of care" (AACN, 2007, p. 6). The accountability and willingness to accept responsibility for the advancement of the nursing profession must be embraced by nursing leaders both in the upper administrative levels and the bedside setting. According to Haase-Herrick and Herrin (2007), "The knowledge that is leveraged, synthesized, and used to provide care is grounded in relationships between the patient and the multi-disciplinary team" (p. 57). Although any individual can engage in evidence-based practice within a clinical setting, the CNL uses leadership and communication skills to facilitate the interdisciplinary team engaged in client care.

When staff nurses were asked the reasons for not embracing research- and evidence-based practice, the challenges identified were the lack of staff understanding about research, the failure to see the usefulness of research in everyday practice, and the disappointment that the questions raised at the bedside were not being answered (Albert & Siedlecki, 2008). Bedside nurses must value the benefits of evidence-based practice while embracing the need to become involved with the process of evidence-based practice. Munroe, Duffy, and Fisher (2008) acknowledged evidence-based practice as an integral component of nursing care "strategies that simultaneously educate, stimulate, and support all nursing staff in identifying clinical nursing questions and searching for evidence-based nursing interventions to address these questions" (p. 55). The CNL is in a pivotal position to marshal the nurse researcher and the questions identified by bedside nurses, thus moving evidence-based practice forward to address the key issues of quality patient care.

According to Melnyk and Fineout-Overholt (2005), evidence-based practice involves five steps: "[ask] the burning clinical question, collect the most relevant and best evidence, critically appraise the evidence, integrate all evidence with one's clinical expertise, patient preferences, and values in making a practice decision or change, and evaluate the practice decision or change" (p. 9). Each step is important to ensure effective and quality implementation of evidence-based practice components. Before asking the question, the CNL should access bedside nurses to engage them in the determination of the critical questions to be addressed within any specific setting. The bedside nurse frequently identifies a principle barrier to evidence-based practice as the lack of perceived value for the concerns they identify within the practice arena. By involving them in the process, interest and commitment to the process can be expected.

Within evidence-based practice, the crucial question is usually formulated using the PICOT structure instead of a hypothesis or research question.

P The *population* to be used. Care should be given to narrow the population as much as possible.

I The *intervention* that is being considered. It does not have to be any actual action but is the care aspect under investigation. For example, the intervention could be listed as the use of alcohol-based, hand sanitation devices for cleaning of hands between patient care activities.

C A *comparison* to another care aspect incorporated into the process. Given the prior intervention example, a comparison could be made with hand-washing with antibacterial soap lasting 20 to 30 seconds between patient care activities. Within the formation of PICOT questions, a comparison does not have to be used in each question; the intervention can stand alone in some questions.

O The expected *outcome*. Each PICOT question is expected to have at least a population, intervention, and outcome determined and incorporated into the question.

T Any *time* limit to be used. The time designation may not be identified as important within some PICOT types of problem identification. For example, if the question relates to the development of postoperative infections, a time limit would become important, but for a question related to use of education to reduce the number of obese children, the time aspect would not necessarily be used.

A narrow, well-developed PICOT question allows a clear direction for collecting evidence that is pertinent to the topic. PICOT-formulated questions can be readily converted to hypotheses or research questions when needed.

Once the PICOT question is established, the investigation into relevant and applicable evidence can begin. The different aspects identified and clarified through the process of determining the population, intervention, comparison, outcome, and time designations are instrumental in directing the database searches. As articles are found that address the aspects included in the PICOT, the critical evaluation of each article can be completed. Many different formats exist for use in appraising articles. Within evidence-based practice, the level of the evidence is a key characteristic of the article that has to be determined. Several different levels of evidence classifications are available for use. The principal facet within the determination of the levels is the research methodology utilized within the research article. Research studies that incorporate an experimental design are a stronger methodology than a quasi-experimental, nonexperimental, or qualitative design.

Once the PICOT question is determined and the level of evidence identified, the challenges move to integrating the evidence with the nurse's expertise and the patient's preferences and values. Although research evidence is critical to the foundation of the evidence-based practice, these other aspects must also be considered and incorporated as appropriate. The use of expertise, preferences, and values allows for the individualization and holistic provision of health care. As a plan of care is determined based upon the material gained about the subject, evaluation of any practice decisions and/or changes must be conducted.

Decision-Making Theories

With the rapid changes in the healthcare arena and the mandate for patient safety from the Institute of Medicine (IOM) and accrediting bodies such as The Joint Commission and nursing organizations such as the American Organization of Nurse Executive (AONE) and AACN, it is imperative that the CNL be cognizant of decision-making theories. Knowing what method the CNL uses to make clinical decisions at the bedside is essential to provide safe, effective patient care. Bucknall (2007) suggested "two cognitive models of decision making: intuition and analysis" (p. 560). The intuition model is a rapid, unconscious weighing of information, whereas the analytical model is slow and systematic. Most nurses have experienced both models. For example, nurses will often enter a patient's room and think, "There is something wrong with the patient." It is an intuitive gut reaction. However, upon reflection the nurse might note that the patient is "fidgeting and picking at the bed linens. Coloring is pale/ashy; respirations are shallow; perspiration is present on the patient's face." This becomes more analytical as the evidence is documented so that a decision to have the rapid response team notified becomes evident.

Jones (2007) indicated that decision making is different from problem solving. Decision making requires identification and selection of a course of action. Problem solving identifies a problem and finds a solution. Decision making is action utilizing a problem-solving process. Jones further discussed the SWOT (*strengths, weaknesses, opportunities,* and *threats*) method of decision making. This approach allows for a matrix approach that focuses on choices related to a goal. Care must be taken to avoid a narrow focus, which would prevent the full opportunity to work out innovative strategies to address the problem identified. Although multiple options for change must be considered, opportunities for mistakes without the fear of penalties must be considered and employed as options are selected.

Tomey (2009) also promoted exploring all alternatives. She suggested that there are five organizational decision-making models:

1. The *rational model* includes common goals, competence, and processes to achieve individual and organizational values.
2. The *political model* involves the elements of power for addressing and considering conflicting values.
3. The *collegial model* involves group consensus and mutual respect for all members in the group.
4. The *bureaucratic model* is the most common and is founded on policy/procedures, history, tradition, and norms of the organization that doesn't recognize political power struggles or informal communication.
5. The *garbage can model* is a serendipitous model based on unplanned change with a chance for repeated mistakes. The model focuses on key player creativity.

The CNL utilizes different methods based on the challenges confronted. Each individual usually has one or two methods that are more comfortable for use but can move between them according to the problem.

Yoder-Wise (2007) proposed four decision-making model theories:

1. *Normative or prescription theory* involves an objective, routine approach to structured problems. Decisions are based on policy and standard procedures.

2. The *descriptive or behavioral theory* is subjective, not routine, and not structured. This includes past experience and group process.
3. The *satisficing model* is a conservative approach that minimally meets a standard. It may be the easiest and quickest approach to a decision.
4. The *optimizing* theory involves making decisions that are based on maximum objectives to meet a standard. This process of looking at pros, cons, benefits, and cost as a decision avenue takes more time but can produce better results.

What Constitutes Evidence?

According to Oman et al. (2008), "Only a small percentage of healthcare professionals incorporate research evidence into clinical decision making" (p. 47). As a result, CNLs need to select a decision-making theory to examine the evidence. The challenge is to decide what constitutes evidence and then to translate the evidence to practice. Albert and Siedlecki (2008) offer a model for evidence-based nursing practice that incorporates a body of evidence (knowledge) translated to practice (policies, procedures, and standards of care) built on quality improvement and research findings.

Stichler (2008) suggested using the Problem/Population (P), Intervention (I), Comparison (C), and Outcomes (O) process for assisting in identifying the evidence for clinical decision making. Stichler offers several sources using various search engines to gather evidence for clinical decisions. Search engines and databases such as Cumulative Index of Nursing and Allied Health Literature (CINAHL), Medline, Embase, PsycINFO, and the Cochrane Database of Systematic Reviews are utilized to locate evidence that can readily present a specific facet of the problem. The more evidence available, the more sound the foundation for the decision.

Kalisch and Curley (2008) offered the SWOT approach for involving new nurses and physicians in a transformation process to allow for nurses to have a major voice in decision making at the unit and organizational levels. Within the effort to transform the workplace, multiple action teams were developed. To further support and develop the transformation, a mentoring program, rapid response team, and Nurse of the Year awards for use of critical thinking and evidence-based practice criteria were instituted to reflect the value of critical thinking and evidence-based practice.

AONE and AACN have combined efforts to develop competencies for the CNL role to include point-of-care decisions based on the best evidence possible (Haase-Herrick & Herrin, 2007; Herrin & Spears, 2007). Rapid change, complexity, and patient safety initiatives require access to the latest evidence for the CNL to provide and manage patient care. To accomplish this, the CNL must receive education and training to gather the most current, valid evidence through a variety of approaches: PICOT, literature searches, research studies, grand rounds, clinical experiences, and patient preferences. Munroe et al. (2008) suggested that "... research findings are evidence for a basis for nursing practice ..." (p. 55). CNLs can use research findings and clinical practice guidelines for evidence to support evidence-based practice. The CNL will need knowledge to appraise and apply that research.

Several depictions of the hierarchy of evidence are available for consideration. Each of the different presentations of levels of evidence identifies and prioritizes the evidence for quality and dependability. Melnyk and Fineout-Overholt (2005) suggested ranking the evidence as follows:

Level 1: Systemic review or meta-analysis of randomized controlled trials and evidence-based clinical practice guidelines

Level 2: One well-designed randomized controlled trial

Level 3: Quasi-experimental studies documented without randomization

Level 4: Well-designed case-control and cohort studies

Level 5: Systematic reviews of descriptive and/or qualitative studies

Level 6: Single descriptive and/or qualitative studies

Level 7: Expert opinion and/or expert committee reports

Each level provides a different attention to the depth of research controls. The hierarchy of evidence provides a means for classifying the research results, but additional items are used to balance evidence-based practice. Although quality evidence is imperative, patient preferences and clinical expertise are placed within the balance as decisions for practice are made.

Appraisal and Application of Research

Health care, thus nursing care, is permeated by chaos and uncertainty (Sanford, 2007). The CNL cannot get away from the puzzlement that is too often imbedded in the healthcare arena. Time and energy is directed toward the movement through the maze of conclusions and evidence placed before the practitioner to establish the quality care issues and practices. According to Herrin and Spears (2007), "It is critical that nurse leaders have the knowledge and competency to develop outstanding relationships with registered nurses in order to retain them and thus improve patient outcomes" (p. 231). By engaging the staff nurses in the challenge of addressing key questions identified within their practice, the benefit of investigating the status quo can be visualized and realized. Albert and Siedlecki (2008) asserted that questions and issues communicated by clinical nurses have the capacity to significantly augment the enhancement of the science and art of nursing. Too often clinical nurses view their questions and issues as not being valued nor addressed. Yet, they are the ones that are in the trenches, doing the hands-on work with individuals who expect and demand quality, innovative attention to their health needs.

An important aspect acknowledged by Layman (2008) is that "health care organizations do not have to discover new nursing interventions to achieve best practice: they simply have to use their resources to discover the evidence that makes best practice" (p. 17). The role of the CNL is to challenge each and every policy and procedure utilized in the clinical setting to determine if it is based on evidence or traditions. The clinical leadership role at the bedside is to confirm that the skills and tasks that are provided are indeed founded on facts and evidence. The challenge of tasks, skills, policies, and procedures does not mandate that things are changed, but only that they are confirmed as correctly conducted using the best knowledge known about the situation. After CNLs confirm the practices employed at a clinical site, they must understand how to communicate the best practices to the required levels of administration. As policies and procedures are identified that require changes, the communication of the rationales for the changes must be based on the evidence.

Ireland (2008) suggested that the evidence-based process should include creating a question, pinpointing associated information, assessing the basis of the information, and appraising the attributes of the information. Each of the aspects within the evidence-based process reflects the strengthening of the rationale for the final intervention, modification, or change resulting. Because CNLs are in a position to identify perspectives from clinicians and administrators, they can identify ways to improve the work environment and patient care. Thus, questions raised by the bedside nurse can be framed by the CNL to facilitate the evidence-based process. Concerns identified by administration can be addressed by the CNL within an evidence-based setting to mesh both levels to ensure quality and safe health care for the client. The CNL is in the position to be able to nurture and cultivate an environment in which staff nurses feel safe to make hunches, raise questions, and seek solutions to complex problems.

Within the complex and confusing healthcare arena, the CNL will be expected to partner with the patient, family, and interdisciplinary members to meet the needs and prospects. These individuals are expected to enter the healthcare setting with multisystem and chronic conditions that interact with acute disease episodes. As the CNL attempts to coordinate the multisystem and chronic conditions aggravated by the acute episode, support systems, available resources, and top-notch health care will tax the CNL to provide the health care grounded on best practices. According to Haase-Herrick and Herrin (2007), "Knowledge about the many aspects of care and emerging evidence will be crucial to professional nursing practice" (p. 56). Being comfortable with accessing the evidence related to the differing nursing practices will be an essential skill demanded of the CNL. The CNL will be required to move from critical thinking to critical synthesis. The utilization of the information via synthesis must be foundational for the CNL engaged in evidence-based practice. Synthesis is the integrated sum total ensuing from the blending of diverse and unique thoughts, influences, or beliefs. Thus, the CNL will incorporate the many differing bits of knowledge, facts, experience, and patient preferences foundational for evidence-based practice that reflects a deeper understanding of the material than is seen in critical thinking.

One method for facilitating the growth and development of evidence-based practice in a healthcare setting is through the use of nursing grand rounds. According to Furlong et al. (2007), nursing grand rounds are intended to "foster advancement of nursing practice by addressing the learning needs of nurses in clinical practice, provide a forum for peers to recognize individuals for clinical expertise, foster networking among diverse clinical nursing specialty areas, and promote the value of each nurse's contribution" (p. 288). Within nursing grand rounds, individuals provide up-to-date research and evidence-based guidelines for discussion. As the individuals discuss the materials presented, the applicability to a unique setting can be determined. The expertise of peers is championed while establishing a level of expectations. Furlong et al. (2007) stated that "the opportunity to share clinical knowledge and experiences beyond the immediacy of daily care" is a means of acknowledging and advocating for the clinical practice of nursing (p. 290). As nurses teach nurses the process of evidence-based practice, the fear of evidence-based practice decreases because colleagues are available to aid and support others as they delve into the process.

Another example of the use of evidence-based practice is evident from the algorithm developed by the University of Colorado Hospital (Oman et al., 2008). Within their Magnet-designated hospital, each policy and procedure is upgraded using the policy and procedure algorithm, which has 10 steps:

1. Select the policy for revision.
2. Search for evidence.
3. Conduct a systematic evaluation of the evidence.
4. Compare evidence to current policy and make a decision.
5. Conduct a policy review by stakeholders/experts.
6. Make revisions based on stakeholders'/experts' comments.
7. Obtain approval signatures.
8. Submit policy to the Patient Care Policy and Procedure Subcommittee.
9. Educate staff as needed.
10. Submit for Web publication.

As each policy and procedure is developed and/or revised based upon this algorithm, the references associated with the process are attached to the document. By including a reference list with the policy and procedure, any individual can quickly see and evaluate the foundation used for that document. Although research-based evidence is highly valued, research is not always available for certain nursing/health interventions. When research results are not found to substantiate a policy or procedure, the amount of evidence becomes the foundation for the recommendations. The more sources of evidence that validate a particular intervention or practice, the more compelling and persuasive the evidence.

Within a study completed by Kalisch and Curley (2008), five steps were identified as useful in transforming a nursing organization: (1) setting the stage for change, (2) management training, (3) strategic planning, (4) developing and implementing changes at the nursing organization level, and (5) developing and implementing changes at the nursing unit level. The logic of using these five steps within any organizational change process reflects thought and attention to the different cultures present within the organization. CNLs work within the microsystem process. The cohesiveness of the cultures at the different levels and buy-in by each and every level within the system are imperative. By carefully and thoughtfully completing a SWOT analysis while working within the restrictions of each level encountered, the outcome for the process can be successful. According to Kalisch and Curley (2008), "Essential ingredients found to be necessary for the success of the project are support from top administration, provision of the necessary resources, willingness to face the brutal facts, early and ongoing attention to sustainability, infusion into the grassroots, unrelenting communication, emphasis on building and maintaining trust, not declaring success too soon, and recognizing that you cannot fully know how" (p. 80). Each of these aspects must be thoughtfully and conscientiously considered.

Having a clear vision from the ground up, and ensuring that the administration understands that vision, is paramount. The CNL holds an important position in bringing both staff members and administration to the table as any project is envisioned and moved forward. The CNL is also in a key position to ensure that sufficient celebrations of intermittent successes are observed effectively. Each and every member within the team needs to commemorate the team's progress toward the goal. Another aspect for the CNL to actively facilitate is the determination of progressive measures and methods of tracking so that the accomplishments can be observed. As noted, Kalisch and Curley (2008) identified that "leadership did not tell managers and staff what to do to achieve excellence but asked the questions that would assist nursing staff and managers to develop answers and provide the data that would help them see alternative ways of functioning, information they could not ignore" (p. 81). The CNL does not do it by him- or herself for the unit, but rather challenges the team to envision every aspect of the project so that the outcome is the team's success, not someone else's. The CNL is a mentor to aid the different members of the team to strive for excellence and to be successful in that endeavor to reach for the stars. Too often staff members feel forgotten or disregarded. When the CNL and administration can be effective partners in championing the staff members, the resulting positive environment is realized in more than just the one unit or on the one shift. The optimistic and constructive culture is established that then can impact many different areas within the healthcare setting.

Outcome Evaluation

Goodman (2003) defined *outcome research* as "the effort to find out whether a particular intervention worked in a particular place" (p. 79). The functionality of outcomes within the process provides a foundation for growth of any profession. Outcomes provide a clear, concise picture of the value of the activities that are being used within management, bedside care, or other key areas within the healthcare setting. One aspect for current discussion is the quality of the evidence. Care must be given to validate the evidence and the quality of the evidence to be used. The CNL can be instrumental in clarifying the level of evidence used within any policy, procedure, or guideline under consideration at a particular site. As a result, the CNL can serve as uniquely positioned gatekeeper in regard to the guidelines and evidence incorporated into policies and procedures. Attention to the quality and dependability of the evidence is necessary. Malloch and Porter-O'Grady (2006) asserted, "Evidence-based practice is not a cookbook or cookie-cutter approach to developing or managing clinical practice. It requires a degree of flexibility and fluidity based on firm scientific and clinical evidence validating appropriate and sustainable clinical practice" (p. 3). The sustainability of the delivery of nursing care is one key aspect that must be consistently understood and considered. If evidence recommends a path that is not sustainable for all settings and all clients, careful consideration of other paths must be investigated. The CNL needs to keep an open mind concerning the delivery of nursing care. Each policy and procedure or guideline necessitates regular review and revision as appropriate based on quality evidence.

According to Morjikian, Kimball, and Joynt (2007), "Whether the proposed intervention is budget-neutral or not, nurse leaders are expected to make a sensible business case for a new practice model, which includes quantitative analysis of cost and benefits along with revenue and expense calculations" (p. 400). The CNL has to prepare and document the analysis that is foundational for any proposed intervention. In addition to a firm understanding of nursing/healthcare issues, the business side must be integrated to support the rationales provided as policies and procedures, clinical interventions, and innovative practice models are championed. The necessary investigation of the evidence to support and defend the rationales is a key aspect that will strengthen the requested modifications. This preliminary work to determine the evidence lends endorsement when done carefully and professionally. As CNLs become effective at getting "all their ducks in a row" before asking for change, the outcomes will have a great chance for success. Taking the time and energy to research the proposed practice changes allows for questions and concerns to be carefully considered and the best plan developed. Smith and Dabbs (2007) stated that the utilization of the CNL skills increases the influence nursing has on health care while making an impact on the quality and safety of patient care through the use of evidence-based practice. This movement to incorporate the CNL results in raising the applicability of nursing as the leader of the healthcare team within a patient-focused manner instead of the outdated, discipline-focused manner.

Taylor and Allen (2007), in their examination of the vision of evidence-based nursing practice, raised several interesting points. Two fundamentally different visions of evidence-based practice—academic and service—are discussed. With the time and workload restrictions perceived by the bedside nurse, the implementation of evidence-based practice becomes a critical aspect. Many schools of nursing are modifying undergraduate research courses to provide an understanding of the process to complete research appraisals. Even graduate programs are seen as modifying research courses to give additional attention to the appraisal aspect. With a strong focus on completing appraisals for incorporation into evidence-based guidelines, the process of conducting research is left to be somewhat learned "on the job." Both the procedural instructions and the appraisal process are critical to the effective movement toward a nursing delivery system that is evidence-based. Someone has to be educated and encouraged to conduct the research so that the evidence can be found and incorporated.

It is also important that the evidence be balanced with patient preferences and experience. Evidence-based guidelines are valuable but must be thoughtfully incorporated based on the setting. The CNL is positioned to carefully and consciously critique the guidelines while aiding the bedside nurse to balance the evidence with client needs and experience. Each aspect—evidence, client needs, and experience—needs to be valued in the application of evidence-based nursing practice.

Conclusion

The call from AACN (2007) for the CNL is the mitigating of clinical measures rooted in evidence while accepting the challenge to seek and utilize evidence that probes current policies and procedures in the practice arena and assimilating evidence into the practice setting, which includes the education of other healthcare team members as necessary. The advancement of the CNL role through the use of evidence-based practice incorporates the strengths of leadership, communication, and validated nursing practice to improve the provision of safe and effective health care for the clients encountered.

Oman et al. (2008) suggested although scientific evidence is embraced by the nursing profession to direct practice and advance outcomes, the day-to-day incorporation of the evidence-based practice process is challenging and overwhelming to the bedside nurse. For the nurse at bedside, practical and efficient methods must be implemented to ensure that the process is manageable and functional in the busy work environment within diverse health settings.

According to Tachibana and Nelson-Peterson (2007), "The implementation of the CNL role has successfully addressed the gap that existed in assuring that patients with complex care needs receive the consistency and continuity of care from a nurse . . . who can articulate the plan of care across shifts and disciplines, improve patient outcomes and satisfaction, and provide resources and expertise to both patients and staff" (p. 479). Although the gap can be bridged by this nursing role, the ultimate outcome is for the improvement of healthcare provision to the clients encountered in a diversity of settings who present with complex, acute, or chronic health challenges.

Tools of the Trade: Case Studies

Case Study 1: Introducing Evidence-Based Practice

Upon being hired as a CNL for an acute care facility in an urban city, one of the first challenges you have is to establish an evidence-based practice climate on the medical/surgical unit to which you have been assigned. The unit is a 50-bed ICU step-down medical/surgical unit. The staff is primarily associate-degree-prepared registered nurses and certified nursing assistants. The core staff members state that they are too overwhelmed to learn anything new. They are just trying to get the job done while providing quality health care for the clients on the unit.

Consider the following questions related to this scenario:

1. What type of information should you collect and assess before making any changes to the unit environment?
2. What types of projects would you think about beginning to introduce evidence-based practice into this medical/surgical unit?
3. How can you best make this change to an evidence-based environment while ensuring that the change is a "win-win"?

Case Study 2: Building a SWOT Team

The hospital in which you are employed has decided to begin the Magnet journey. As a result, the CNLs have been given the challenge to determine a plan for implementing evidence-based practice within the facility. What steps would the CNL team need to use to conduct a SWOT (strength, weakness, opportunities, and threats) analysis?

Consider the following questions related to this scenario:

1. What type of considerations must be made as a SWOT analysis is initiated?

2. How can the team of CNLs identify strengths, weaknesses, opportunities, and threats for the implementation of evidence-based practice?

3. What types of projects might be used to engage the staff in completing the SWOT and implementing a plan?

Case Study 3: Decision-Making Methods

Multiple decision-making methods exist for an individual to use. Effective decision making is the goal of the process. Consider the different decision making theories listed. In what settings would the different decision making theories work best?

Consider the following questions related to this scenario:

1. Compare the advantages and disadvantages of using intuition or analysis in making decisions. Which method would work best in an emergency setting? Which method would work best in an outpatient setting?

2. In what type of settings does the SWOT method of decision making tend to work best? Why?

3. Considering the five organizational decision making models identified by Tomey (2009), which ones do you feel most comfortable using and why?

Summary

- CNLs have the responsibility and expectation to make a difference not only in the acute care setting but across the healthcare delivery spectrum. In all settings in which nursing leaders are engaged in the delivery of health care to individuals, families, or community, the obligation to incorporate sound and tested health practices is essential.

- No longer can the nursing profession depend on "that's how we have always done it" as a reason for providing substandard health care to the public. Every skill and task undertaken within the realm of nursing should be supported by evidence.

- The accountability and willingness to accept responsibility for the advancement of the nursing profession must be embraced by nursing leaders both in the upper administrative levels and the bedside setting.

- A narrow, well-developed PICOT question allows a clear direction for evidence collecting that is pertinent to the topic.
- Decision making requires identification and selection of a course of action. Problem solving identifies a problem and finds a solution. Decision making is action utilizing a problem-solving process.
- The hierarchy of evidence provides a means for classifying the research results, but additional items are used to balance evidence-based practice. Although quality evidence is imperative, patient preferences and clinical expertise are balanced as decisions for practice are made.
- The CNL is in the position to be able to nurture and cultivate an environment in which staff nurses feel safe to make hunches, raise questions, and seek solutions to complex problems.
- When the CNL and administration are effective in championing the staff members, the resulting positive environment is felt in more than just one unit or on one shift. The optimistic and constructive culture is established that then can impact many different areas within the healthcare setting.
- The advancement of the CNL role through the use of evidence-based practice incorporates the strengths of leadership and communication, and validates nursing practice to improve the provision of safe and effective health care for the clients encountered.

Reflection Questions

1. What type of clinical questions have you heard discussed on the medical unit by bedside personnel? How have you encouraged this dialogue to address the issues, problems, and challenges identified within the provision of health care?
2. Consider the different policies and procedures that are used at your facility. How much and what level of evidence was used in the establishment of these documents?

Learning Activities

1. Pull four to five nursing/medical journal articles. Assess the level of evidence reflected within each article. On the basis of this review of the articles and the level of evidence, is the material presented appropriately and documented for use within the practice of nursing?

References

Albert, N. M., & Siedlecki, S. L. (2008). Developing and implementing a nursing research team in a clinical setting. *Journal of Nursing Administration, 38*(2), 90–96.

American Association of Colleges of Nursing (AACN). (2007). *White paper on the education and role of the clinical nurse leader.* Washington, DC: Author.

Boswell, C., & Cannon, S. (2007). *Introduction to nursing research: Incorporating evidence-based practice.* Sudbury, MA: Jones and Bartlett.

Bucknall, T. (2007). A gaze through the lens of decision theory toward knowledge translation science. *Nursing Research, 56*(Suppl. 4), S60–S66.

Furlong, K. M., D'Luna-O'Grady, L., Macari-Hinson, M., O'Connel, K. B., Perez, E. L., & Pierson, G. S. (2007). Implementing nursing grand rounds in a community hospital. *Clinical Nurse Specialist, 21*(6), 287–291.

Goodman, K. W. (2003). *Ethics and evidence-based medicine: Fallibility and responsibility in clinical science.* Cambridge, UK: Cambridge University Press.

Haase-Herrick, K. S., & Herrin, D. M (2007). The American Organization of Nurse Executives' guiding principles and American Association ot Colleges of Nursing's clinical nurse leader. *JONA, 37*(2), 55–60.

Herrin, D., & Spears, P. (2007). Using nurse leader development to improve nurse retention and patient outcomes: A framework. *Nursing Administration Quarterly, 31*(3), 231–243.

Ireland, M. (2008). Assisting students to use evidence as a part of reflection on practice. *Nursing Education Perspectives, 29*(2), 90–93.

Jones, R. A. P. (2007). *Nursing leadership and management in nursing: Theories, processes, and practices.* Philadelphia: F. A. Davis.

Kalisch, B. J., & Curley, M. (2008). Transforming a nursing organization: A case study. *JONA, 38*(2), 76–83.

Layman, E. L. (2008). Implementing evidence-based nursing practice. *Nurse Leader, 6*(1), 15–17.

Malloch, K., & Porter-O'Grady, T. (2006). *Introduction to evidence-based practice in nursing and health care.* Sudbury, MA: Jones and Bartlett.

Melnyk, B. M., & Fineout-Overholt, E. (2005). *Evidence-based practice in nursing and healthcare: A guide to best practice.* Sudbury, MA: Jones and Bartlett.

Morjikian, R. L., Kimball, B., & Joynt, J. (2007). Leading change: The nurse executive's role in implementing new care delivery models. *Journal of Nursing Administration, 37*(9), 399–404.

Munroe, D., Duffy, P., & Fisher, C. (2008). Nurse knowledge, skills, and attitudes related to evidence-based practice: Before and after organizational support. *MEDSURG Nursing, 17*(1), 55–60.

Oman, K. S., Duran, C., & Fink, R. (2008). Evidence-based policy and procedures: An algorithm for success. *Journal of Nursing Administration, 38*(1), 47–51.

Sanford, K. (2007). Confronting the perfect storm: A challenge to nurse leaders. *Nursing Administration Quarterly, 31*(2), 120–123.

Schoenfelder, D. P. (2007). Simply the best: Teaching gerontological nursing students to teach evidence-based practice. *Journal of Gerontological Nursing, 33*(8), 6–11.

Smith, D. S., & Dabbs, M. T. (2007). Transforming the care delivery model in preparation for the clinical nurse leader. *Journal of Nursing Administration, 37*(4), 157–160.

Stichler, J. F. (2008). Finding evidence to support facility design decisions. *Journal of Nursing Administration, 38*(4), 153–156.

Tachibana, C., & Nelson-Peterson, D. L. (2007). Implementing the clinical nurse leader role using the Virginia Mason Production System. *Journal of Nursing Administration, 37*(11), 477–479.

Taylor, S., & Allen, D. (2007). Visions of evidence-based nursing practice. *NurseResearcher, 15*(1), 78–83.

Tomey, A. M. (2009). *Guide to nursing management and leadership* (8th ed.). St. Louis, MO: Mosby-Elsevier.

Yoder-Wise, P. S. (2007). *Leading and managing in nursing* (4th ed.). St. Louis, MO: Mosby-Elsevier.

NINE

Nursing Informatics for the Clinical Nurse Leader

■ Ramona Nelson, Christine Meyer, and Bonnie B. Anton

■ **Learning Objectives**

■ Analyze the implications of current trends in the development of health-care information systems.

■ Discuss the relationship between nursing informatics and the CNL.

■ Participate in the selection and implementation of healthcare information systems.

■ Identify resources supporting the effective use of automation in health care.

> "Where is the wisdom we have lost in knowledge? Where is the knowledge we have lost in information?"
>
> T. S. Eliot

Key Terms

Barcode-enabled point-of-care technology (BPOC)

Clinical decision support (CDS)

Computerized provider order entry (CPOE)

Consumer informatics

Electronic health record (EHR)

Health information exchange (HIE)

Health literacy

Health Insurance Portability and Accountability Act (HIPAA)

Nursing informatics

Personal health record

CNL Roles

Information manager

Outcomes manager

Member of a profession

Team member

System analyst and risk anticipator

Client advocate

Educator

CNL Professional Values

Altruism

Integrity

Social justice

Accountability

Human dignity

CNL Core Competencies

Information and healthcare technologies

Nursing technology and resource management

Human care systems and policy

Communication

Assessment

Introduction

Throughout the history of humankind, society has been impacted by the development of technology. Today the technical tools of automation are changing many aspects of modern society including all aspects of healthcare delivery. A major factor influencing the roles, functions, and success of CNLs is the automation of healthcare delivery. The CNL assumes a number of roles, particularly related to information and technology.

For example, as an outcome manager, the CNL understands and synthesizes the data, information, knowledge, and wisdom model in managing clients and in working with other members of the healthcare team. As a client advocate, the CNL actively encourages the development of an empowered consumer of healthcare services and information. This includes patient education concerning effective and safe use of the Internet and personal health records. The CNL as educator ensures that clients and providers receive proper education and training to effectively use information systems in health care. As an information manager, the CNL effectively uses the tools of automation in the management of both clinical and administrative data. This includes the effective and appropriate use of decision support systems. The CNL in the role of systems analyst/risk anticipator understands and prevents e-iatrogenesis errors. Assuming the role of team manager, the CNL effectively uses the concepts inherent in the life cycle to participate in the selection and implementation of healthcare information systems that support quality, safe patient care, and the practice of the CNL. Lastly, as a member of a profession and lifelong learner, the CNL accesses and uses informatics-related professional associations as a resource in making informatics-related decisions and in maintaining a current understanding of the role informatics plays in healthcare delivery.

CNL Core Professional Values and Information and Technology Management

Using information and technology, core professional values ground the CNL in best use of the data and processes. The value of altruism illustrates the CNL's demonstration of the importance of building information systems that are sensitive to the beliefs, cultures, and values of both providers and patients. Accountability, as a core value, considers the use of automated information systems to collect and utilize evidence needed for evidence-based practice. The CNL demonstrates the value of human dignity by balancing patient privacy rights with the information needs of clinicians for access to patient data and information. Integrity, as a value, ensures that data maintained in current healthcare information systems are current, accurate, and comprehensive. The CNL's core value of social justice promotes legislation and policy related to the use of information systems in health care that ensures universal access while providing for patient privacy. This requires an understanding of current trends and innovations.

Given this reality, CNLs must be prepared to play a key role in directing that change. As a professional group and as individual professionals they are responsible for ensuring that automated healthcare delivery systems are designed to support healthcare practitioners provide effective, efficient, and quality patient care. This chapter introduces information and skills a CNL needs to meet this responsibility. This includes an understanding of nursing informatics (NI), an understanding of the major trends in healthcare technology driving the automation of the healthcare system, and an appreciation of the life cycle of a healthcare information system and CNL responsibilities.

CNL Core Competencies in Information and Technology Management

Each of the core competencies of a CNL is absolutely essential in using automated systems to complete the roles of a CNL. In today's healthcare settings, information systems are utilized to manage patient and institutional data, information, and knowledge. Wisdom is the appropriate use of data, information, and knowledge to manage all aspects of patient care and healthcare delivery. In order to make effective decisions and provide quality care, a CNL must (1) identify what nursing data should be included in a healthcare information system, (2) determine how data should be processed to produce pertinent nursing information, (3) apply nursing knowledge in interpreting data and information, and finally (4) utilize nursing wisdom in using an automated system to support evidence-based practice as a CNL.

Understanding Data and Information

Data are raw facts without meaning or interpretation. For example, the number 120 could be a diastolic or systolic blood pressure, or the weight of a thin, 6-foot-tall male or an obese third-grader. Without context or interpretation the number has no meaning. Many nursing students begin their education learning how to assess a patient by collecting appropriate data elements. Novice staff nurses soon learn to collect all of the important patient data before jumping to conclusions. Likewise, novice CNLs soon learn to collect all of the key facts before reaching an administrative decision.

Information is a collection of data that has been processed and interpreted to produce meaning. For example, data could be used to graph the relationship between patient-staff ratios and patient satisfaction. The information (meaning) contained within the line graph is determined by the knowledge of the person reading the graph. For example, a CNL would pull upon his or her knowledge of factors that influence patient satisfaction and ask additional questions about the level of staff, the acuity of the patients, the type of clinical unit, and so forth.

The use of the words *information* and *knowledge* in everyday conversation demonstrates the difference between these two concepts. For example, visitors to a hospital would check with the *information desk*, not the knowledge desk. On the other hand, a teacher may refer to a student as having a good *knowledge base* in a specific area. As a general rule, the novice will tend to remember facts or information, whereas the expert becomes skillful in identifying the interrelationships.

Wisdom is the appropriate use of knowledge, information, and data in solving real-life problems. It involves the use of empirical, ethical, personal, and esthetic knowledge combined with values and experience. For example, a CNL may be able to list and explain the stages of grief and dying, but be uncomfortable talking to a client about his or her terminal illness. A CNL may not remember the details of these stages, but may have an intuitive feel for where the client is and how to talk with the client about the terminal illness. A CNL will have an intuitive sense of how to support a new staff member in their first year of nursing and only vaguely remember reading the details of reality shock. These details have now been integrated into an overall gestalt that guides the intuitive sense of what to do when.

Trends Driving Healthcare Technology

The belief that the American healthcare delivery system is broken, is forcing both government and private groups to act. Health care has been described as fragmented, unaffordable, and often unsafe. "The frustration levels of both patients and clinicians have probably never been higher. Yet the problems remain. Health care today harms too frequently and routinely fail to deliver its potential benefits" (IOM, 2001). Increasingly, an empowered consumer is demanding a safe, secure healthcare delivery system that is affordable for all Americans. This demand can be as simple as the elderly person who asks, why do I have to walk half way across the campus of a major medical center to register as a patient before I can have a simple blood draw done in a different area? Or it can be as complex as the patient who has reviewed several articles in MEDLINE and questions why her treatment is inconsistent with published standards of practice. For many, the solution is effective implementation of information technology throughout the healthcare system.

The focus of the federal government's efforts can be seen in the several "key topics" identified on the Agency for Healthcare Research and Quality Health IT home page (http://www.ahrq.gov). At the top of the list are (1) the electronic medical/health records with access to a national health information exchange (HIE), (2) electronic prescribing including computerized provider order entry (CPOE) and barcode medication administration, and (3) providing for the security of healthcare information.

Information Tools and the CNL

Electronic Health Records Patient safety is perhaps the most cited reason to implement an EHR. Medical errors are a major threat to patient safety. "To Err Is Human: Building a Safer Health System," published in 1999 by the Institute of Medicine, proposed that there are between 44,000 and 98,000 preventable deaths each year in the United States primarily due to medical errors (IOM, 1999). A common denominator underlying these errors is faulty systems that permit the errors to occur in the first place. This report recommended that the healthcare industry examine these faulty processes and develop strategies that would assist individuals to perform the correct action. The implementation of an electronic clinical system plays a significant role in reducing the cost of health care, reducing complications, and achieving better outcomes (Amarasingham, Plantinga, Diener-West, Gaskin, & Powe, 2009).

Integral to the establishment of comprehensive patient records is a process for sharing clinical data across hospital boundaries. This process is now supported by the federal government in the form of a health information exchange (HIE). HIE refers to the sharing of clinical and administrative data across the boundaries of healthcare institutions and other health data repositories. Many stakeholder groups, from payers to providers, realize that if such data are shared safety, then quality, cost, and other indicators of healthcare excellence would be improved. With this goal in mind, the Nationwide Health Information Network (NHIN) is being developed to provide a secure, nationwide, interoperable health information infrastructure connecting providers, consumers, and others involved in healthcare delivery. This critical part of the national health IT agenda will enable health information to follow the consumer, be available for clinical decision making, and support appropriate use of healthcare information beyond direct patient care (U.S. Department of Health and Human Services, Health Information Technology, n.d.).

The need for an efficient, affordable, and safe healthcare delivery system has also motivated private groups. An important example of private groups driving healthcare reform through the use of technology is the Leapfrog Group. A significant portion of the healthcare costs in the United States are covered by employers who purchase healthcare insurance for their employees. The Leapfrog Group is a consortium of major companies and other large private and public healthcare purchasers who are providing health benefits to more than 37 million Americans in all 50 states. This voluntary group is aimed at utilizing employer purchasing power to alert the health industry that improvement in healthcare safety, quality, and customer value will be recognized and rewarded.

An important factor in any implementation project is to obtain ongoing input from users. The CNL plays a pivotal role in eliciting their ideas for establishing the content, screen displays, and the clinicians' role. Representatives from each medical specialty review the paper order sets and agree on the contents of each order set for their respective specialty. Requests to create orders sets for individual physicians such as "Dr. Smith's Admission Orders" are strongly discouraged in an effort to adhere to guidelines and to decrease patient care variability (Fisher, Creusat, and McNamara, 2008).

The Informed, Empowered Consumer
Historically, consumers have, for the most part, played a passive role in influencing healthcare delivery. However, as access to information has improved and out-of-pocket expenses have increased, this is changing. Increasingly, consumers are using the Internet to educate themselves about their healthcare problems and options and to compare quality and costs. With the proliferation of health information, CNLs are able to communicate with patients electronically in their home setting, which has great potential to reduce patient admissions and readmissions.

Privacy and Electronic Health Records The privacy and security of an electronic record is a major concern for providers and patients alike. In 1996 Congress passed a federal law known as the Health Insurance Portability and Accountability Act (HIPAA) to achieve the following:

- Provide Americans with greater access to health insurance
- Promote national standards for code sets, such as CPT-4 and ICD-9 Diagnosis Codes, for the electronic transfer of health data

- Protect the privacy of health data (U.S. Department of Health and Human Services, 2006)

As a CNL, it is important to assume a leadership and advocacy role in understanding the importance of maintaining patient privacy.

The Healthcare Information System

When an organization selects a healthcare information system, the CNL plays an important role in collecting information from staff and stakeholders and providing information about the benefits and risks of the system. A tool that CNLs may use during this process includes the following phases:

1. Identify the stakeholders and staff.
2. Review the information system benefits and risks.
3. Develop an information flyer of benefits and risks.
4. Establish an implementation team.
5. Assist with piloting the system.
6. Train the staff.
7. Assist with evaluating the system and planning for future applications.

Summary

- Nursing informatics is the specialty that integrates nursing science, computer science, and information science to manage and communicate data, information, knowledge, and wisdom in nursing practice (ANA, 2008).
- Professional organizations in nursing informatics can provide CNLs with knowledgeable professional contacts and new opportunities to learn about healthcare technology.
- The ultimate goal of a national EHR is universal access to one's medical records anywhere and anytime with built-in safeguards to ensure data privacy and security.
- Increasingly, empowered consumer are taking a direct hand in understanding their health problems, their treatment options, and maintaining electronic records related to their health care.
- CNLs must assume a leadership role throughout the life cycle of a healthcare information system.

Reflection Questions

1. Will the adoption of an electronic health record create a totally paperless chart?
2. What are the advantages and disadvantages of a totally paperless medical record? Does "paper kill"? See the following URL to frame your answer: http://www.providersedge.com/ehdocs/ehr_articles/Paper_Kills_Should_Be_Healthcare-s_Mantra.pdf.
3. What are the implications of a terrorist attack on electronic health records? What are the implications of a natural disaster, such as Hurricane Katrina, on paper records?
4. Should the electronic medical records be hosted by individual healthcare institutions, by individual patients, or by both?
5. Should the selection of health information systems be controlled by experts in the information technology department?
6. Should health teaching done by staff nurses routinely include a review of safe Internet practices?
7. Does automation increase or decrease the security of health records?
8. How does the informed, empowered patient redefine the patient-provider relationship?
9. What implications do automatic healthcare information systems have for the development of standard nursing languages?

Learning Activities

1. Spend the day learning about electronic systems, particularly documentation and data tracking methods in your microsystem. Write a 3- to 5-page paper on your major findings.
2. Using the information from Learning Activity 1, "crosswalk" one process within the system—for example, admitting a patient, discharging a patient, or performing a patient procedure. Identify successes and failures from this exercise. Did you observe patterns or trends?

Recommended Reading

Agency for Healthcare Research and Quality. (2005). *30 safe practices for better health care: Fact sheet.* AHRQ Publication No. 05-P007. Retrieved February 14, 2009, from http://www.ahrq.gov/qual/30safe.htm

American Cancer Society (ACS). (2008). *Finding support*. Retrieved February 26, 2009, from http://www.cancer.org/docroot/MBC/content/MBC_4_1X_Finding_Support.asp?sitearea=MBC

American Health Information Management Association (AHIMA), e-HIM Personal Health Record Work Group. (2005, July–August). The role of the personal health record in the EHR. *Journal of AHIMA, 76*(7), 64A–D. Retrieved February 26, 2009, from http://library.ahima.org/xpedio/groups/public/documents/ahima/bok1_027539.hcsp?dDocName=bok1_027539

American Medical Informatics Association (AMIA). (n.d.). *About AMIA*. Retrieved February 23, 2009, from http://www.amia.org/inside

American Nurses Credentialing Center (ANCC). (n.d.). *Certification*. Retrieved February 7, 2009, from http://www.nursecredentialing.org/Certification.aspx

American Nursing Informatics Association. (n.d.). *About ANIA*. Retrieved February 26, 2009, from http://www.ania.org/About%20ANIA.htm

Anderson, H. J. (2009, January 1). *CPOE: It don't come easy*. Retrieved February 8, 2009 from http://www.healthdatamanagement.com/issues/2008_60/27494-1.html

Arnold, S., Wagner, J., Hyatt, S. J., Klein, G. M., & Global EHR Task Force Members. (2007). *HIMSS: Electronic health records; A global perspective*. Retrieved October 8, 2007, from http://www.himss.org/content/files/DrArnold20011207EISPresentationWhitePaper.pdf

Audet, A., Doty, M. M., Peugh, J., Shamasdin, J., Zapert, K., & Schoenbaum, S. (2004). Information technologies: When will they make it into physicians' black bags? *Medscape General Medicine 6*(4), 2.

Averbeck, B. M. (2005, November). Bringing evidence-based best practices into practice. *Health Management Technology, 26*(11), 20, 22. Retrieved October 7, 2007, from http://archive.healthmgttech.com/archives/1105/1105bringing_evidence.htm

Berner, E. S., Detmer, D. E., & Simborg, D. (2005). Will the wave finally break? A brief view of the adoption of electronic medical records in the United States. *Journal American Medical Informatics Association, 12*, 3–7. Retrieved September 29, 2007, from http://www.cms.hhs.gov/SecurityStandard/Downloads/SecurityGuidanceforRemoteUseFinal122806.pdf

Blum, B. (1986). *Clinical information systems*. New York: Springer-Verlag.

Bush, G. W. (2004, April 30). Executive Order 13335: Incentives for the use of health information technology and establishing the position of the national health information technology coordinator. Retrieved February 12, 2009, from http://edocket.access.gpo.gov/2004/pdf/04-10024.pdf

Campbell, E. M., Sittig, D. F., Ash, J. S., Guappone, K. P., & Dyskstra, R. H. (2006). Types of unintended consequences related to computerized provider order entry. *Journal of American Medical Informatics Association, 13*(5), 547–556.

CARING. (n.d.). *About CARING*. Retrieved February 26, 2009, from http://www.caringonline.org/mc/page.do?sitePageId=29212

Centers for Medicare & Medicaid Services (CMS). (2008). *E-prescribing overview*. Retrieved February 19, 2009, from http://www.cms.hhs.gov/eprescribing

Citizen's Council on Health Care. (2008, October 22). *National patient ID would violate patient privacy rights*. Retrieved February 14, 2009, from http://www.cchconline.org/pr/pr102208.php

eHealth Initiative. (2008). *Electronic prescribing: Becoming mainstream practice*. Retrieved February 12, 2009, from http://www.ehealthinitiative.org/assets/Documents/eHI_CIMM_ ePrescribing_Report_6-10-08_FINAL.pdf

Fioriglio, G., & Szolovits, P. (2005). Copy fees and patient's rights to obtain a copy of their medical records: From law to reality. *AMIA 2005 Symposium Proceedings,* 251–255. Retrieved September 28, 2007, from http://www.pubmedcentral.nih.gov/articlerender.fcgi?artid=1560890

Fox, L. A. (2004). Health record paradigm shift: Consumer health informatics. *2004 IFHRO Congress & AHIMA Convention Proceedings.* Retrieved February 20, 2009, from http://library.ahima.org/xpedio/groups/public/documents/ahima/bok3_005546.hcsp?dDocName=bok3_005546

Fox, S. (2006). *Online health search 2006*. Retrieved February 22, 2009, from http://www. pewinternet.org/Reports/2006/Online-Health-Search-2006.aspx

Goedert, J. (2009, January 8). Obama: EHRs for all in five years. *Health Data Management.* Retrieved February 12, 2009, from http://www.healthdatamanagement.com/news/NHIN27526-1.html

Graves, J., & Corcoran, S. (1989). The study of nursing informatics. *Image: The Journal of Nursing Scholarship, 21*(4), 227–230.

Hagen, S. (2008). *Estimating the effects of health IT on health care costs* (Congressional Budget Office). Retrieved February 12, 2009, from http://www.himss.org/advocacy/d/ 2008PublicPolicyForumHandouts/StuartHagen.pdf

Halamka, J. (2006). The perfect storm for electronic health records. *Journal of Health Care Information Management, 20*(3), 25–27. Retrieved October 26, 2007, from http://www.himss.org/content/files/08_column_ehr.pdf

Healthcare Information Management Systems and Society (HIMSS). (n.d.a). *About HIMSS.* Retrieved February 20, 2009, from http://www.himss.org/ASP/aboutHimssHome.asp

Healthcare Information Management Systems and Society (HIMSS). (n.d.b). *Chapters represent the grassroots of HIMSS!* Retrieved February 20, 2009, from http://www.himss.org/ASP/chaptersHome.asp

Healthcare Information Management Systems and Society (HIMSS). (n.d.c). *CPHIMS certification.* Retrieved February 26, 2009, http://www.himss.org/ASP/certification_cphimsAbout.asp

Healthcare Information Management Systems and Society (HIMSS). (2007). *EHR: Electronic health record.* Retrieved October 5, 2007, from http://www.himss.org/ASP/topics_ehr.asp

Healthcare Information Management Systems and Society (HIMSS). (2009). *Advocacy news: Healthcare reform update: This week's view from the executive branch.* Retrieved February 22, 2009, from http://www.himss.org/advocacy/contentredirector.asp?contentid=68956

Hillestad, R., Bigelow, J. H., Chaudhry, B., Dreyer, P., Greenberg, M. D., Meili, R. C., et al. (2008). Identity crisis: An examination of the costs and benefits of a unique patient identifier for the U.S. health care system [Monograph]. Retrieved February 14, 2009, from http://www.rand.org/pubs/monographs/2008/RAND_MG753.pdf

Jha, A. K., Dollan, D., Grandt, D., Scott, T., & Bates, D. W. (2008). The use of health information technology in seven nations. *International Journal of Medical Informatics, 77*(12), 848–854.

Leape, L. L., Bates, D. W., Cullen, D. J., Cooper, J., Demonaco, H. J., Gallivan, T., et al. (1995). Systems analysis of adverse drug events. ADE prevention study group. *JAMA, 274*(1), 35–43.

The Leapfrog Group. (2007). *The Leapfrog Group fact group.* Retrieved October 13, 2007, from http://www.leapfroggroup.org/media/file/leapfrog_factsheet.pdf

National Association of Chain Drug Stores. (2007). *Industry facts-at-a-glance.* Retrieved February 13, 2009, from http://www.nacds.org/wmspage.cfm?parm1=507

National Institutes of Health National Center for Research Resources. (2006). *Electronic health records overview.* Retrieved October 7, 2007, from http://www.ncrr.nih.gov/publications/informatics/EHR.pdf

National League for Nursing (NLN). (1988a). *Preparing nurses for using information systems: Recognized informatics competencies.* New York: Author.

National League for Nursing (NLN). (2008b, May 9). *Preparing the next generation of nurses to practice in a technology-rich environment: An informatics agenda.* Retrieved February 20, 2009, from http://www.nln.org/aboutnln/PositionStatements/informatics_052808.pdf

National Network of Libraries of Medicine. (2008) *Health literacy.* Retrieved February 23, 2009, from http://nnlm.gov/outreach/consumer/hlthlit.html

Nebeker, J. R., Hoffman, J. M., Weir, C. R., Bennett, C. L., & Hurdle, J. F. (2005). High rates of adverse drug events in a highly computerized hospital. *Archives of Internal Medicine, 165*(10), 1111–1116.

Nelson, R. (2002). Major theories supporting health care informatics. In S. Englebardt & R. Nelson (Eds.), *Health Care Informatics: An Interdisciplinary Approach.* St Louis, MO: Mosby.

Nelson, R., & Joos, I. (1989). On language in nursing: From data to wisdom. *PLN, 1*(5), 6.

Nielsen-Bohlman, L., Panzer, A. M., & Kindig D. A. (Eds.). (2004, April 8). *Health literacy: A prescription to end confusion.* Washington, DC: National Academies Press.

Privacy Rights Clearinghouse. (2007). *Fact sheet 8(a): HIPAA basics: Medical privacy in the electronic age.* Retrieved September 22, 2007, from http://www.privacyrights.org/fs/fs8a-hipaa.htm

Rogoski, R. R. (2002). The ABCs of CPRs and EMRs. *Health Management Technology.* Retrieved October 7, 2007, from http://archive.healthmgttech.com/archives/h0502abc.htm

Saba, V. K., & McCormick, K. A. (2006). *Essentials of computers for nurses: Informatics for the new millenium* (4th ed.). New York: McGraw-Hill.

Schillinger, D., Grumbach, K., Piette, J., Wang, F., Osmond, D., Daher, C., Palacios, J. (2002, July 24–31). Association of health literacy with diabetes outcomes. *JAMA, 288*(4), 475–482.

Upham, R. (2004). *The electronic health record: Will it become a reality?* [HIPAA Advisory]. Retrieved September 30, 2007, from http://www.hipaadvisory.com/action/ehealth/EHR-reality.htm

U.S. Department of Health and Human Services. (2008). *CMS improves patient safety for Medicare and Medicaid by addressing never events.* Retrieved February 12, 2009, from http://www.cms.hhs.gov/apps/media/press/factsheet.asp?Counter=3224&intNumPerPage=10&checkDate=&checkKey=&srchType=1&numDays=3500&srchOpt=0&srchData=&keywordType=All&chkNewsType=6&intPage=&showAll=&pYear=&year=&desc=false&cboOrder=date

U.S. Department of Health and Human Services, Office for Civil Rights. (n.d.). *Personal health records and the HIPAA Privacy Rule*. Retrieved February 22, 2009, from http://www.hhs.gov/ocr/privacy/hipaa/understanding/special/healthit/phrs.pdf

U.S. Department of Health and Human Services, Office for Civil Rights. (2009a). *Resolution agreement: CVS pays $2.25 million & toughens disposal practices to settle HIPAA privacy case*. Retrieved February 20, 2009, from http://www.hhs.gov/ocr/privacy/hipaa/ enforcement/examples/cvsresolutionagreement.html

U.S. Department of Health and Human Services, Office for Civil Rights. (2009b). *Frequently asked questions about the disposal of protected health information*. Retrieved February 23, 2009, from http://www.hhs.gov/ocr/privacy/hipaa/enforcement/examples/disposalfaqs.pdf

van Uden-Kraan, C. F., Drossaert, C. H., Taal, E., Seydel, E. R., & van de Laar, M. (2008). Self-reported differences in empowerment between lurkers and posters in online patient support groups. *Journal of Medical Internet Research, 10*(2), 1–18.

Weiner, J. P., Kfuri, T., Chan, K., & Fowles, J. B. (2007). "e-Iatrogenesis": The most critical unintended consequence of CPOE and other HIT. *Journal of American Medical Informatics Association, 14*(3), 387–388.

References

Amarasingham, R., Plantinga, L., Diener-West, M., Gaskin, D. J., & Powe, N. R. (2009). Clinical information technologies and inpatient outcomes. *Archives of Internal Medicine, 169*(2), 108–114.

American Nurses Association (ANA). (2008). *Scope and standards of nursing practice*. Silver Spring, MD: Author.

Fisher, S. R., Creusat, J., & McNamara, D. (2008). *Improving physician adoption of CPOE systems: Lessons learned from the field*. [White paper]. Retrieved August 4, 2008, from http://www.strategiestoperform.com/docs/ImprovingPhysicianAdoption.pdf

Institute of Medicine (IOM). (1999). *To err is human: Building a safer health system*. Washington, DC: National Academies of Science.

Institute of Medicine (IOM). (2001). *Crossing the quality chasm: A new health system for the 21st century*. Washington, DC: National Academy of Sciences.

U.S. Department of Health and Human Services. (2006). *HIPAA security*. Retrieved October 27, 2007, from http://www.cms.hhs.gov/SecurityStandard/Downloads/SecurityGuidanceforRemoteUseFinal122806.pdf

U.S. Department of Health and Human Services, Health Information Technology. (n.d.). *Health information exchange: Background*. Retrieved February 26, 2009, from http://healthit.ahrq.gov/portal/server.pt?open=514&objID=5554&mode=2&holderDisplayURL=http://prodportallb.ahrq.gov:7087/publishedcontent/publish/communities/k_o/knowledge_library/key_topics/health_briefing_01232006093812/health_information_exchange.html#Background1

Unit 4

Community Resource Awareness and Networking Through Advocacy

TEN

Community Resource Awareness and Networking Through Advocacy

■ Linda Roussel, Alice J. Godfrey, and Lonnie Williams

■ **Learning Objectives**

- ■ Describe the CNL's roles as patient advocate and community leader.
- ■ Evaluate tools used in discharge planning and community diagnosis.
- ■ Outline creative tools for team building and collaboration.
- ■ Identify community outreach and networking opportunities for the CNL.

> "Never doubt that a small group of thoughtful committed citizens can change the world, indeed it's the only thing that ever has."
>
> **Margaret Mead**

Key Terms

Discharge planning

Community outreach

Community diagnosis

Social justice

CNL Roles

Outcomes manager

Educator

Systems analyst and risk anticipator

Client advocate

Information manager

Team manager

CNL Professional Values

Accountability

Social justice

Human dignity

CNL Core Competencies

Communication

Nursing technology and
    resource management

Disease prevention

Ethics

Designer/manager/
    coordinator of care

Assessment

Health promotion

Risk reduction

Information and healthcare technologies

Human care systems and policy

Introduction

The clinical nurse leader (CNL), as the designer, manager, and coordinator of care, provides and assembles comprehensive care for clients: individuals, families, groups, and communities, in multiple and varied settings. According the American Association of Colleges of Nursing (AACN), the CNL guides the patient through the health systems using skills essential to this role. Such skills include communication, collaboration, negotiation, delegation, coordination, and evaluation of interdisciplinary work, and the application, design, and evaluation of outcome-based practice models (pp. 25–26).

Preparation of the CNL

Preparing the CNL for community resource management and networking includes course work in leadership, interdisciplinary team building, organizational skills, information management, delegation, and cost-benefit analysis. The CNL considers the environment's readiness for change and processes important to that end. Understanding organization and community culture, how decisions are made, and key stakeholders in translating best practices provides the CNL with skill sets to accomplish these goals. The CNL does not work alone. Creating a vision for the stakeholders with those at the point of care (patients, family, staff, multidisciplinary teams, and community members) helps to spread and sustain quality and safe care. Patient involvement in their care, working to facilitate decision making and self-management, is strengthened when involving interdisciplinary teams and community networks.

Leadership and Interdisciplinary Team Building

As a horizontal leader, the CNL is key to the healthcare team, serving as a critical navigator through the microsystem. The CNL knows the roles of the various team members and the value they add to the safe passage of the patient into the community. The CNL understands concepts of team building and the skills necessary to build quality teams. Such skills include visioning, group dynamics, accountability, and basics on how to conduct a meeting. Complexity science advances concepts for the larger view of social systems and community networking, important knowledge for the CNL to possess.

Complexity and Community Networking

Complexity theory provides new insights into the behavior and emergent properties of social systems. Complexity theory purports that the experience of community is both an outcome and the context of *informal networking*. A well-connected community is achieved when people feel part of a web of diverse and *interlocking relationships*. These networks sustain and shape an integrated and dynamic social and organizational environment. They support the familiar patterns of interaction and collective organization that characterize the voluntary and community sectors. Community development involves creating and managing opportunities for connection and communication across sectoral identity and geographical boundaries. Termed *meta-networking*, it is a core function of the professional role. The community can be envisioned as part of the microsystems when the population of patients at the microsystem level is cared for within this system. Failing to take into consideration where patients are going (and coming from), and the neighborhood and community support available creates a fissure in the system. This underscores the silos that health care continues to reinforce, often related to reimbursement methods.

The professional values of the CNL support his or her active involvement with the community. When assuming responsibility for the comprehensive care of individuals, families, and population groups, the CNL participates in the care of the communities in which their clients live, work, and play. The CNL advocates for the worth and value of all persons and individualizes a plan for continuity of care that reflects a commitment to the principle of social justice. Social justice considers the CNL's responsibility for fair, equitable care. Competency in providing health care to diverse populations and working with diversity is also integrated into social justice.

Discharge Planning

Discharge planning is a concept that has long been recognized as essential in the delivery of quality health care. The process rose to the forefront in healthcare management with the passage of legislation that mandated it as an essential service. Today, discharge planning is a critical process that requires interdisciplinary teamwork. The identification of healthcare resources, as well as evaluation of these resources, is essential to the implementation of the CNL's role.

The key features of the discharge planning process are as follows:

- Planned and coordinated events in any patient care setting
- Contribution to the continuity of patient care services
- Promotion of health maintenance and safety of patients as they access and consume healthcare services
- Contribution to the cost-effectiveness of healthcare services
- An interdisciplinary process

Networking and Discharge Planning

The CNL will identify the persons in the clinical microsystem who contribute to the process. Some of the individuals may be directly involved with the patient. These individuals include the physician, nurses, social worker, therapists, and laboratory providers. However, administrative support is critical for policies to be implemented effectively.

Tools Used in Discharge Planning

Discharge planning begins with the first encounter with the patient. The individual patient assessment tools will include information about the patient's diagnosis as well as living arrangements, family, and significant others. Each microsystem will have standard tools for patient assessments. Information obtained in the patient's initial assessment serves to direct the CNL to tools that will assist with the identification of discharge needs as well as diagnosing community needs. Two tools that will contribute to the success of discharge planning and community diagnosis are the epidemiologic triad and the natural history of disease model.

The Epidemiologic Triad

Disease in humans is typically explained in terms of the *epidemiologic triad*, which is a tool that is central to community diagnosis.

The epidemiologic triad describes the complex interaction of the human host with a disease-causing agent and the environment in which the interaction occurs. Host characteristics can be such factors as age, sex, race, religion, customs, occupation, previous disease, and immune status. Types of disease-causing agents may include biologic, bacterial, viral, chemical, and nutritional. Temperature, humidity, altitude, crowding, food, water, air pollution, and noise are identified environmental factors that can cause an increased risk of human disease. It is the interaction of these factors (host, agent, environment) that contributes to disease. Analysis of the host characteristics, possible agents, and environmental factors enable the CNL to identify risks that can contribute to the onset of disease and disability. According to Gordis (2009), disease can be caused by biologic, physical, chemical factors. Psychosocial factors also contribute to disease occurrence but may not fit into the usual categorization of factors.

The Natural History of Disease Model

The natural history of disease model is a classic tool by Leavell and Clark (1965). The model describes the progression of disease. There are two disease periods in this model: the prepathogenesis period and the pathogenesis period. The prepathogenesis period begins with the interaction of host, agent, and environmental factors. As disease develops in the person, the model includes the phases of pathogenesis that the person experiences. The levels of prevention are correlated to the periods of prepathogenesis and pathogenesis (primary, secondary, and tertiary). Primary prevention focuses on the prepathogenesis period, whereas secondary and tertiary prevention focus on the pathogenesis period. Primary prevention considers health promotion and may include such interventions as health education; provision of adequate housing, recreation, and working conditions; and periodic selective examinations. Primary prevention related to specific protection can be protection against occupational hazards, accidents, and carcinogens; use of specific nutrients; and avoidance of allergens. Secondary prevention related to early diagnosis, prompt treatment, and disability limitation includes such interventions as case finding measures, screening surveys, and adequate treatment to arrest the disease process and prevent further complications and contraindications. Tertiary prevention is included in the period of pathogenesis. Rehabilitation is central to tertiary prevention. Provision of hospital and community facilities for retraining and education for maximum use of remaining capacities describe important interventions in rehabilitation (tertiary prevention). Additional rehabilitation interventions may include education of the public and industry to utilize the rehabilitated, selective work placement and work therapy in hospitals. This model offers a blueprint for health promotion as well as disease management in individuals and at the community level. For example, the CNL who documents an increase in young males who are injured in motorcycle accidents will investigate primary prevention strategies for preventing accidents at the community level. A community diagnosis emerges when the absence of a needed service or the presence of an agent that contributes to disease is identified at the community level.

Community Diagnosing: CNL Role

Tools to Guide Creative Discharge Planning and Community Continuity

Mind Maps can provide an excellent tool in leading teams through innovation. According to Buzan (2004), Mind Maps give depth and breadth of scope that a list of ideas cannot. "By working from the centre outwards, Mind Map encourages your thoughts to behave in the same way" (p. 8). The framework provides an illustrative view of your ideas and their expansion and alternatives, radiating creative thinking. By using letters and numbers, colors and images, Mind Maps engage the left and the right sides of the brain. Starting from the center, working outwardly with ideas, symbols, colors, numbers, and other symbols engages thinking power that increases synergetically. "Each side of the brain simultaneously feeds off and strengthens the other in a manner which provides limitless creative potential" (p. 9). Mind Maps are useful for short- and long-term planning. Working with teams can be more efficient when employing Mind Maps. They can help your team focus on the way ahead and bring together a shared, creative, and imaginative vision. Techniques include incorporating equal time to listen and speak; showing interest in people and ideas; and having a clear idea of where you, the team, and the organization are all headed.

For example, using Mind Maps, focus the team on the core of your innovation, then, using brainstorm sessions, work out specific strategies and ideas. Revisit the Mind Maps as ideas are advanced or carried out, with new options surfacing with the changes. The Mind Map can serve as an agenda, a business plan, and as the basis for developing project plans. Considering this nonlinear (complexity) way of thinking, Mind Maps offer a natural way to innovate.

Buzan also offers TEFCAS (trial, event, feedback, check, adjust, and success) as a success mechanism for working with Mind Maps. Each aspect of this mechanism identifies tools, a checklist, and strategies for applying a different way of thinking. TEFCAS helps to monitor and react to the outcome of project plans, focusing on goals and outcomes. This model reinforces project planning, adding new insights to ongoing processes.

The Use of Story: Messages to Innovate Team Collaboration

Loehr (2007) described the power of story as a means of changing one's destiny in business and in life. Loehr shared the following:

> By "story," then, I mean those tales we create and tell ourselves and others, and which form the only reality we will ever know in this life. Our stories may or may not conform to the real world. They may or may not inspire us to take hope-filled action to better our lives. They may or may not take us where we ultimately want to go. But since our destiny follows our stories, it's imperative that we do everything in our power to get our stories right. (p. 5)

Bringing about ways to understand your story and that of your organization can be critical to understanding the mission and goals to be carried out. Knowing your own story (about success, challenges, and use of opportunities and challenges) is a good place to start. Reflecting on your values and beliefs, the "private voice" in your head is part of self-awareness and self-reflection necessary to helping others to understand their story and mutually creating one for the team. Loehr identifies three rules of storytelling: purpose, truth, and action. *Purpose* considers the motives and overall intention of the story. What are we driving for? What principle? What end? What goal? What do we want to see at the end of our day, year? Is the story taking us where we want to go? What is nonnegotiable? These are questions that can guide clarity of purpose (Loehr, 2007, p. 138). A shared vision through story can engage head and heart. *Truth* relates to the authenticity of the story. "Is it grounded in objective reality as fully as possible; that is, does it coincide with generally agreed-upon portrayal of the world? Or is it true only if I'm living in a dreamland?" (p. 138). Being truthful gives credibility to leading innovation in patient care delivery. *Action* relates to the purpose and the truthfulness of the story being told. "Does the story move others to action?" Knowing how explicit actions (plan) will be played out for desired outcomes, can provide a dynamic template for the team. This action plan involves the stakeholders, their engagement in the process and outcomes, and how the story plays out.

Stories engage the heart and the mind. The CNL can use story to bring alive what may seem like static processes, policies, and procedures that may be considered mechanistic and carried out in robotic fashion.

Equipped with knowledge and skills in discharge planning, community outreach, and creative collaboration, the CNL furthers the business case for safe, quality continuity of care. Effective discharge planning through a greater understanding of community outreach, networking, and tools such as Mind Maps and story can improve financial, quality, safety, and satisfaction outcomes as teams come together.

Tools of the Trade: Case Studies

Case Study 1: Individual Level

A 21-year-old pregnant woman who has a history of IV drug abuse is admitted through the emergency department. As the CNL on the labor and delivery unit, you admit the patient and begin the initial assessment and discharge planning. Consider the following questions as the discharge planning begin.

1. Who does the patient consider her family?
2. Where does the patient currently live, and where will she go when she leaves the hospital?
3. What personal, environmental, and safety concerns will the patient have when she leaves the hospital?
4. What health and medical follow-up care will she need?

5. After considering questions 1–4, use the natural history of disease model to identify primary, tertiary, and prevention interventions that the patient might need.

Case Study 2: Community Level

Examine the histories and assessment data of the patients on your unit or microsystem. Focus on the demographic profiles of the patients. Do the patients come from one community or neighborhood? Are the patients referred by primary providers or by another agency, such as a nursing home or home care agency, or are they admitted through the emergency department? Are patients being discharged back to the same setting, or are they referred to another level of care?

1. Describe your microsystem's discharge, and consider the referral and support resources used. Do you observe any patterns? If so, what are the patterns?
2. Describe your microsystem's follow-up plan for patients. If the follow-up plan includes contact with the patients after discharge, describe that process.
3. How does your microsystem evaluate the discharge process and its effect on the patient and community? Is there a method of documenting outcomes?

Strategies for Continuity of Care

The CNL will demonstrate leadership, as well as creativity, in the provision of continuity of care. Development of strategies requires interdisciplinary communication, prioritization skills, and community assessment skills. Community assessments identify resources and gaps in services in the community. Anderson and McFarlane (2000) identified eight elements of a comprehensive community assessment:

1. Physical environment
2. Recreation
3. Education
4. Economics

Box 10-1 Example of Community Outreach Assignment

This assignment gives you the opportunity to evaluate community services, referrals, and other community resources that your patients/consumers access in your clinical microsystem. You are asked to consider patient discharge planning and how patients on your unit (in your microsystem) use community services (your major referral support services). In the same vein, where are patients being admitted from (in your community)? What patterns are you seeing regarding admissions and discharges? In other words, are patients coming from the same communities and settings (home, nursing homes, senior centers, etc.)? Are patients being discharged back to their same settings? What have you learned from this assignment?

_____/3 points: Describe your microsystems' discharge plan considering referral and support sources. Do you observe any patterns? If so, what are the patterns?

_____/3: Outline primary sources and follow-up plans. Do you have contact with your patients after discharge? If so, describe the continuity of care and how this impacts the quality and safe delivery of services and patient satisfaction.

_____/3: Outline recommendations to improve community outreach and ongoing continuity of patient care.

_____/1: APA, Material is in APA style, has a scholarly presentation, and uses reference citations liberally

_____/10%/10%

5. Communication
6. Health and social services
7. Politics and government
8. Safety and transportation

Any service or resource considered for a patient needs to be evaluated. The questions in Box 10-2 can serve as a guide when evaluating community resources.

Box 10-2   Evaluating Community Resources

- Is the agency an official or governmental agency?
- Is the agency a private or voluntary agency?
- What is the level of prevention addressed by the services of the agency?
- What are the eligibility requirements for the service?
- What are the cost of services, and what payment sources are accepted?
- How are referrals made?
- How are families and significant others included in the services provided?
- What is the preparation and expertise of the service provider?

Case Study 3: Leadership and Advocacy in the Community

Assessment of the patient data, as well as the discharge planning process in your microsystem, reveals the following information.

A significant number of patients with type II diabetes have been admitted over the last year. The patients reside in the zip code where a new retirement community that provides housing for low income persons over age 65 has just been established. The patients have different primary care providers. The neighborhood is on the public bus route that will transport residents to a chain grocery and shopping center.

1. Who would you consider to be stakeholders in this neighborhood?
2. How would you go about initiating a diabetic management clinic for the retirement community?

Summary

- As reimbursement tightens with greater demands for efficient, effective care, discharge planning and community networking have greater criticality.
- The CNL in the role of outcomes manager, client advocate, and team manager provide an understanding of quality improvement data, using evidence-based practice methods to promote a smooth transition of care from setting to setting.

- As an educator, information manager, systems analyst, and risk anticipator, the CNL uses tools for discharge planning and community diagnosing, including the epidemiologic triad and the natural history of disease model.
- Additional strategies include Mind Maps and story, which contribute to engaging staff and communicating and collaborating with teams.
- CNL core competencies—such as communication, assessment, nursing technology and resource management, health promotion, and risk reduction—are essential to CNL success in community outreach with patient-centered care.
- Core competencies also include integrating disease prevention, information and healthcare technologies, ethics, and human care systems.

Reflection Questions

1. As a CNL, how do you determine the best strategies to network with community partners?
2. Are there best communication strategies to begin the dialogue with community leaders and stakeholders?

Learning Activities

As a CNL on a fast-based surgical-orthopedic unit, you have noted that after most of your patients are discharged into their community, they often return just weeks later. You note that many of the patients require after-hospital care, including home health services, support groups, long-term care, and assisted living services. Other services, such as Meals on Wheels, medication assistance programs, and assistance with durable medical equipment, are also important to your patients' discharge planning. You begin to see a pattern emerge that there are inadequate resources within your community. You have also noted that your hospital has programs that may be useful to the community.

1. As an outcomes manager, what specific outcomes would be appropriate for you to address the above issues?
2. What are the advocacy issues? As a client advocate, what are your responsibilities? How are these evaluated?
3. As an educator and information manager, how would you determine educational needs and how would you manage this information?

4. As systems analyst/risk anticipator, how would complexity theory guide you in managing community resources?
5. Who would need to be at the "table" as you serve as a team manager?

Recommended Reading

Bourgeault, I. L., & Mulvale, G. (2006). Collaborative health care teams in Canada and the USA: Confronting the structural embeddedness of medical dominance. *Health Sociology Review, 15*(5), 481–494.

Hagenow, N. (2003). Why not person-centered care? The challenges of implementation. *Nursing Administration Quarterly, 27*(3), 203–207.

Summers, L., Marton, K., Barbaccia, J., & Randolph, J. (2000). Physician, nurse, and social work collaboration in primary care for chronically ill seniors. *Archives of Internal Medicine, 160*(12), 1825–1833.

Virginia Regional Medical Program. (1974). *Discharge planning*. Richmond, VA: Author.

References

Anderson, E. T., & McFarlane, J. M. (2000). *Community as partner: Theory and practice in nursing* (3rd ed.). Philadelphia: Lippincott.

Buzan, T. (2004). *Mind Maps at work: How to be the best at your job and still have time to play*. New York: Penguin Group.

Gordis, L. (2009). *Epidemiology* (4th ed.). Philadelphia: W. B. Saunders.

Leavell, H. F., & Clark, E. G. (1965). *Preventive medicine for the doctor in his community: An epidemiologic approach*. New York: McGraw-Hill.

Loehr, J. (2007). *The power of story*. New York: Simon and Schuster.

ELEVEN

Health Policy, Ethics, and Advocacy

■ **Elizabeth Furlong**

■ **Learning Objectives**

- ▪ Describe the CNL's role in health policy, ethics, and patient and professional advocacy.
- ▪ Demonstrate an understanding of how health policy, ethics, and advocacy integrate with one another.

> "If I am not for myself, what am I? If I am only for myself, who am I?"
>
> Jewish proverb

Key Terms

Health policy   Ethics advocacy

CNL Roles

Client advocate   Team manager
Lifelong learning   Member of a profession

CNL Professional Values

Altruism   Accountability
Human dignity   Integrity
Social justice

CNL Core Competencies

Critical thinking   Communication
Illness and disease management   Ethics
Human diversity   Global health care
Member of a profession   Manager of care
Healthcare systems and policy   Designer/manager/coordinator of care
  provider

Introduction

Clinical nurse leaders (CNLs) can best promote quality patient care by integrating health policy, ethics, and advocacy in nursing interventions. This chapter is structured by focusing on 10 strategies of patient advocacy. Integrated with these strategies are concepts of health policy and ethics. It is beyond the purview of this chapter to be comprehensive in a presentation of all three of these issues (health policy, ethics, and advocacy). As the reader will note, the case studies integrate these three issues. It is impossible to unlink their integration. It is the strong commitment of this writer that the CNL has the clinical, professional, moral, ethical, and legal obligations to be involved in health policy and patient advocacy. Nurses are reminded of that commitment from a variety of ethical sources—ethical principles, the American Nurses Association Code of Ethics, and the social contract of nursing with society.

Patient Advocacy

CNLs can use several strategies to advocate for patients. Selected strategies are discussed here. One aspect of advocacy is ensuring continuity of care for the patient population for whom the CNL has responsibility. This will entail the CNL developing collaborative constructive relationships with all institutional representatives in practice—in other words, social workers, physicians, discharge planners, home health agency nurse liaisons, and other nursing staff. The method of "hands-off" communication strategies between nurses of two different shifts in hospitals and/or between nurses of two different institutions varies across the country (Mascioli, Laskowski-Jones, Urban, & Moran, 2009). For example, within an institution, this communication may be face-to-face or physical rounding with each other. The CNL should consider the strategy of physically rounding with the institutional staff nurse or the nurse representative from the agency to which the patient is being transferred. If the patient is being discharged home with a plan of care for a home health nurse for a designated time period, the ideal strategy would be inviting and scheduling the respective home health nurse or home health agency hospital liaison nurse to physically round with the CNL. This should be done with family members also present in the patient's room. In implementing this strategy, the CNL would be "bringing back" to nursing practice a successful patient care strategy used three decades ago.

The CNL uses evidence-based practice (EBP) during daily nursing interventions and in interdisciplinary work as an advocacy strategy. Current literature recommends hourly rounding with patients and specific communication techniques (use of touch, introduction of self, and active listening) as forms of advocacy grounded in the research evidence. Individuals seeking to become a CNL may have experience and trust their knowledge of nursing history and their personal clinical experience and knowledge. They may be at varying levels according to the Benner model of novice to expert (2001). CNLs analyze their strengths and build upon these strengths of clinical decision making and knowledge development. They reflect and recognize parallels over time. For example, hourly rounding with patients, although done routinely 30–50 years ago, was resurrected as a best practice in the past several years. Patient care will be enhanced by the nurse knowing both 21st-century EBP and some core nursing interventions.

Networking also can be considered a strategy of advocacy. The ability of a CNL to provide timely and quality care to patients is directly related to an extensive network of colleagues—both internal and external to the institution. The CNL is attentive to developing and sustaining relationships with all colleagues. Most individuals are cognizant of the importance of the adage, "It not what you know, but, who you know." Knowing a unit secretary well, having a collaborative relationship with a physician, engaging in a respectful relationship with a housekeeper, and being trusted by a respiratory therapist can all reap quality patient outcomes when one utilizes this social capital that has been intentionally developed and sustained. Equally important is to develop relationships with health providers and other organizations outside of the hospital for continuity of care and for knowledge of community resources for patient care.

"Having a voice" is also a strategy of advocacy. The nursing profession rightfully prides itself on the consistent recent number of years in which it has been voted the most trusted profession in the Gallup poll; there is, however, a shadow side to this honor. Buresh and Gordon, feminist journalists, have critiqued nurses and provided examples of how nurses can move from their silence to "having voice" (2006). This has special significance for the CNL who will be one of the leaders in hospitals and other organizational settings. The CNL must "have voice" with administrators, the public media, legislators, and other organizations in advocating for the best care for populations of patients. Although there are several ways to accomplish this, the next example will relate to the specific CNL role. The CNL can be prepared with a "two-minute elevator story" in which others can be educated about the CNL role. In preparing the anecdote, a picture can be painted, jargon avoided for the layperson, facts and statistics included, personal interventions described, and a description of the whole context provided. Creating anecdotes and stories is imperative for the CNL given the newness of the role and the possible misconceptions about it that the public and health providers may have.

Commitment to lifelong learning about the history of nursing advocacy, possible conflicting advocacy models, and emerging theories is another advocacy strategy. Although Hamric (cited in Hanks, 2005) espouses that advocacy is a relatively new role for nursing that emerged in the United States in the 1980s, this may be debated. What can be noted are past degrees of nursing advocacy reflecting the greater societal norms related to class and gender issues (physician and nurse relationships). Further, this level of nursing advocacy reflected the types of communication and problem resolution present in a healthcare system and in a society. This is significant given the level of knowledge diffusion we now have of negotiation and alternative dispute resolution.

Gadow, a nurse ethicist, has contributed much to the nursing literature on patient advocacy (1980). Hanks (2005) has expanded the work with a sphere of nursing advocacy model in which the following is posited. First, the nurse provides a protective shield for the patient with the external environment. Second, the nurse facilitates the patient's self-advocacy. And third, both may simultaneously advocate. This model is built on certain assumptions: (1) only patients can decide what is in their best interest, (2) nurses have moral obligations to enhance a patient's autonomy, (3) nurses must not let their biases interfere with their patient advocacy, and (4) nurses cannot doubt their actions for patients. The CNL can best improve patient outcomes by keeping current on both new theoretical and EBP advocacy interventions.

Intervening as a policy activist is another strategy of advocacy. Boswell, Cannon, and Miller stated it best in their article "Nurses' Political Involvement: Responsibility Versus Privilege" (2005). The authors argue that policy and political involvement is a responsibility; it is not simply a privilege for one's choice of participation or nonparticipation. Their model includes three stages of involvement—survival, success, and significance. The first stage, survival, includes the policy-shaping behaviors of voting, working for candidates, serving on community boards, and registering voters. The next level, success, will have the CNL involved in the following—being a candidate, being a spokesperson for a group, or being an advisor to an elected official. Finally, the third stage, significance, includes these policy-shaping behaviors—assuming strategic leadership positions in healthcare facilities and professional and community organizations—and being a visionary to solve health system problems.

The above is not a comprehensive list of all ways one may be involved in the health policy process, nor is it the only model that one might use. However, it is one way of viewing the policy stances that CNLs need to take. To reiterate, policy activism is a responsibility, not a privilege. This policy activist strategy of advocacy integrates with the American Nurses Association Code of Ethics—as do all the advocacy strategies.

Awareness of the many organizational resources available to CNLs is another advocacy strategy. One example is the partnership between the American Nurses

Association (ANA) and the Healthcare Improvement Initiative in the Saving 100,000 Lives Campaign. This has now been expanded to the 5 Million Lives Campaign (*5 Million Lives Campaign,* 2009). CNLs can take leadership advocacy positions within their respective institutions and participate in this initiative.

Being cognizant of the many ethical dilemmas that present for patients, family members, nursing staff, interdisciplinary health providers, and the CNL is yet another advocacy strategy. Many nurses experience *moral distress,* defined as "knowing what is ethically appropriate but being unable to act on it because of obstacles inherent in a situation" (Chen, 2009, p. 2). The CNL applies knowledge of ethical theories, ethical decision-making processes, and the situational context (power dynamics, conflict in values among decision makers, etc.), and uses institutional resources such as ethics committees. Further, the CNL integrates the aspect of "having voice" versus retreating behavior (nonadvocacy for patients, silence, anger, diminished personal integrity, burnout, etc.).

CNLs are knowledgeable of the traditional ethical principles of nonmalfeasance, beneficence, autonomy, and distributive justice. They may use these principles for decision making, or they may use theories that emerged in the latter decades of the 20th century, for example, an ethic of care. The ethic of care is based on work by feminists and nurses and is more inclusive of the context and situation of the ethical dilemma than the traditional ethical principles listed above (Furlong, 2004). This has been ascribed to the research on gender differences in moral decision making that finds women to be more concerned with relationships and context. Thus, their moral decisions differ from those of men, who use more of a linear justice model.

McSteen and McAlpine (2006) noted that nurses who are professionally competent, have high self-esteem and courage, and engage in risk-taking behaviors are moral agents and advocates. They then extrapolate that such nurses struggle less with moral distress. But advocacy is not simply about having knowledge in the ethical dimension. It also must include attentiveness to one's communication skills, one's approach to conflict, knowledge of power variables in the work setting, knowledge of group dynamics, and so forth. Further skills that CNLs develop include the processes and techniques used in alternative dispute resolution, mediation, and negotiation (Gerardi, 2006). Some strategies of mediation include (1) listening for understanding, (2) reframing, (3) elevating the definition of the problem, and (4) making clear agreements (Gerardi, 2004).

Practicing cultural humility versus cultural competency and modeling this behavior with all staff is an important advocacy strategy. Tervalon and Murray-Garcia (as cited in Hunt, 2001) define *cultural humility* as "a lifelong process of self-reflection and self-critique" (p. 3). To be culturally humble means not learning lists of behaviors about people of different cultures; but, rather, it means being intentional in engaging partnerships with patients to learn their unique priorities, goals, and challenges. This advocacy strategy is especially important for the CNL in this rapidly shrinking global community in which we live.

Another advocacy strategy is the CNL's ability to "see the big picture" and to be part of solving the "big picture" need. This may extend beyond the group of patients for which she cares. For example, in late 2008 and 2009, large numbers of Americans lost their jobs, their health insurance, and their savings. This has created ripple effects in hospitals, healthcare systems, employment opportunities for health providers, wellness and illness behaviors by patients and nonpatients, and so forth. The CNL has broader advocacy, policy, and ethical obligations to society than to a group of 6–10 patients for direct illness care. This obligation must extend to being a part of a solution to such current societal problems. This can take many forms, and CNLs can best assess what they can do in the situation. Poverty and inadequate income were major correlates of illness and promoted this legislation.

The patient advocacy strategies described provide value-added information and will prove useful for successful CNL practice and preparation of students in any practice setting. The following case studies further provide useful examples of how health policy, ethics, and advocacy are integrated.

Tools of the Trade: Case Studies

Case Study 1: Nurses and Health Policy

An example of a nurse participating in health policy involves the promotion of health status of patients with mental illness in a community setting. A CNL may contact a state senator and encourage the introduction of a legislative bill related to patients' needs. This may increase access to mental health services in rural areas. By developing, nurturing, and sustaining relationships with professional organizations, the CNL is a participant in health policy. CNLs will learn of needs experienced by populations of patients that can best be met by legislative change at the state or national level. It is expected that they be patient advocates by initiating, strategizing, lobbying, and championing bills to fruition to meet patient needs. It is not enough to advocate for patients one at a time when one has the knowledge base that the same problem affects entire populations of patients.

Case Study 2: The Power Inherent in a Specialty Nursing Organization

Nurses who belong to the American Nephrology Nurses Association (ANNA) have demonstrated the power of a specialty nursing organization in the combined area of health policy, ethics, and advocacy. Because of their clinical expertise, they noted the negative impact of limited Medicare and Medicaid funding on patients with end-stage renal disease (ESRD). They lived their organization's value of advocacy and clinical excellence by initiating a grassroots advocacy program in 2003 to educate both state and federal lawmakers on ESRD funding issues. They educated 62 policymakers or their aides in 29 states in 2003 with this initiative. Since then, they have educated 350 more such policymakers. Further, because of this, they have experienced some positive federal legislative outcomes for patient funding (Kuchta, VanBuskirk, & Houglum, 2007).

Although the Web site for the Clinical Nurse Leader Association (CNLA) does not specifically list health policy or legislative activity in its mission, vision, or goals statements, it is anticipated that such activities will be added to the association's activities as it matures (Clinical Nurse Leader Association, 2009). The CNLA does partner with the American Association of Colleges of Nursing, which has major active health policy and legislative initiatives. The example given in Case Study 2 can easily be replicated by the CNLA when its members recognize patient needs that can best be met by health policy change—whether it be at the state or the federal level.

Box 11-1   The Intervention Model

For the CNL practicing nursing in the community setting, an opportunity exists to use the intervention model when working with a group of individuals or families (Keller, Strohschein, Lia-Hoagberg, & Schaffer, 2009). This model, which includes 17 public health interventions that can be used with patients, has been extensively studied since the Minnesota Department of Health introduced it in 1998. It is now used throughout the United States and has been subjected to rigorous review by both regional and nursing experts. Advocacy is one of the interventions.

Box 11-2   Advocacy Skills

- Networking skills
- Lobbying skills
- Knowledge of the legislative process
- "Having voice"

Summary

- It is important that the CNL connect to the community and referral sources. Network! Network! Network!
- The CNL is an advocate, working with patients, families, and providers at the point of care delivery. Have voice!
- As an extension of advocacy, the CNL becomes politically involved knowing that being at the table can make a difference and change things for the better. Be a policy activist!
- CNLs can be the change in the healthcare system given the competencies and roles of a lateral integrator, leader, and advocate.

Reflection Questions

1. Reflect on a situation in which you did not "have voice." What would you do differently in a similar situation?
2. If you are not involved in policy-shaping behaviors, what are your barriers?

Learning Activities

1. Participate in some type of policy-shaping behavior that you have not engaged in before.
2. Network in an intentional manner with someone you do not know.

References

Benner, P. (2001). *From novice to expert*. Upper Saddle River, NJ: Prentice Hall.

Boswell, C., Cannon, S., & Miller, J. (2005). Nurses' political involvement: Responsibility versus privilege. *Journal of Professional Nursing, 21*(1), 5–8.

Buresh, B., & Gordon, S. (2006). *From silence to voice*. Ithaca, NY: ILR Press.

Chen, P. W. (2009, February 5). When doctors and nurses can't do the right thing. *The New York Times*. Retrieved May 14, 2009, from http://www.nytimes.com/2009/02/06/health/05chen.html

5 million lives campaign. (2009). Retrieved February 24, 2009, from http://www.nursing world.org/MainMenuCategories/ThePracticeofProfessionalNursing/PatientSafetyQuality/Advocacy/5-Million-Lives.aspx

Furlong, E. (2008). Health care for some borne on the back of the poor. In M. deChesnay & B. A. Anderson (Eds.), *Caring for the vulnerable* (pp. 527–538). Sudbury, MA: Jones and Bartlett.

Gadow, S. (1980). Existential advocacy: Philosophical foundation of nursing. In S. Spicker & S. Gadow (Eds.), *Nursing: Images and ideals* (pp. 79–101). New York: Springer.

Gerardi, D. (2004). Using mediation techniques to manage conflict and create healthy work environments. *AACN Clinical Issues, 15*(2), 182–195.

Gerardi, D. (2006). Team disputes at end-of-life: Toward an ethic of collaboration. *Permanente Journal, 10*(3), 43–44.

Hanks, R. G. (2005). Sphere of nursing advocacy model. *Nursing Forum, 40*(3), 75–78.

Hunt, L. M. (2001). Beyond cultural competence: Applying humility to clinical settings. *Bulletin of the Park Ridge Center for Health, Faith, and Ethics, 24*. Retrieved February 24, 2009, from http://www.parkridgecenter.org/ Page1882.html

Keller, L. O., Strohschein, M. S., Lia-Hoagberg, B., & Schaffer, M. A. (2009). Population-based public health interventions: Practice-based and evidence-supported. *Public Health Nursing, 21*(5), 453–468.

Kuchta, K., VanBuskirk, S., & Houglum, M. (2007). Helping patients with end-stage renal disease [Electronic version]. *AJN, 107*(5), 35–36.

Mascioli, S., Laskowski-Jones, L., Urban, S., & Moran, S. (2009, February). Improving handoff communication. *Nursing, 39*(2), 52–55.

McSteen, K., & McAlpine, C. P. (2006). The role of the nurse as advocate in ethically difficult care situations with dying patients. *Journal of Hospice and Palliative Nursing, 8*(5), 259–268.

Wilson, D. R., Kauzlarich, S. A., & Jensen, L. (2009, February 23). Midlands voices: Mental drug bill adds to subtract. *Omaha World Herald.* Retrieved February 24, 2009, from http://www.omaha.com/index.php?u_page=3952&u_sid=10571223

Unit 5

Health Promotion and Disease Prevention Essentials for the CNL

TWELVE

CNL Role in Health Promotion and Disease Prevention

■ **Barbara M. Carranti**

■ **Learning Objectives**

> "Health is a state of complete physical, mental and social well-being and not merely the absence of disease or infirmity."
>
> **World Health Organization**

- ■ Define health, wellness and illness, and health promotion.
- ■ Compare and contrast health promotion and health protection.
- ■ Discuss the *Healthy People 2010* indicators and how health promotion strategies contribute to the achievement of national healthcare goals.
- ■ Describe the role of the clinical nurse leader (CNL) in health promotion and disease prevention.
- ■ Analyze the role of patient and family education as a health promotion and disease prevention strategy.
- ■ Define health literacy and discuss its importance in promoting health and preventing disease.
- ■ Discuss the impact of culture in promoting health and preventing disease.

Key Terms

Health

Wellness

Health policy

Health protection

Illness

Health promotion

Health literacy

Disease prevention

CNL Roles

Clinician

Outcome manager

Team manager

Educator

Client advocate

Lifelong learner

CNL Professional Values

Altruism

Human dignity

Social justice

Accountability

Integrity

CNL Core Competencies

Communication

Health promotion

Disease prevention

Illness and disease management

Healthcare systems and policy

Designer/manager/coordinator
of care

Assessment

Risk reduction

Human diversity

Provider and manager of care

Member of a profession

Introduction

The leadership role of the CNL is built on generalist clinical knowledge and the ability to integrate care to achieve quality patient outcomes. Health promotion requires knowledge of health regimens, wellness programs, risk assessment and reduction, evidence-based health practices, and safe, effective care. Successful health promotion and disease prevention incorporate knowledge and cultural sensitivity to the client and the ability to formulate tools that can be understood by the client population.

This chapter explores the concepts of health promotion and disease prevention from both the theoretical and application views. Discussion will focus on the health goals of the United States and how health promotion efforts can assist in achievement of these goals. Lifestyle influence on the development of major diseases and life quality are discussed, as well as the economic impact of unhealthy behaviors. Patient and family education is examined as a strategy for assisting with implementation of healthy habits.

Healthcare issues facing Americans at the beginning of the 21st century are largely preventable problems addressed through alterations in lifestyle and environment. Using the *Healthy People 2010* (U.S. Department of Health and Human Services [USDHHS], 2000) data as a barometer, issues such as smoking, substance abuse, and nutritional concerns around obesity, as well as lack of physical activity, have been identified as leading indicators of improvement of the nation's health; these lifestyle factors can be adequately addressed as a part of routine health care. Yet, these issues will often result in acute or chronic health problems that cause hospitalization or other unexpected encounters with the healthcare system.

The CNL can have an impact on lifestyle alterations that can promote health and prevent disease. This generalist has advanced education in health assessment, pharmacology, and pathophysiology, as well as a clinical immersion experience that can assist patients to identify lifestyle and risk factors. As hospital stays shorten, the ability of the CNL to address lifestyle factors contributory to disease risk are critical. The CNL is integral in partnering with patients in their self-management of acute and chronic illnesses. Motivational interviewing is one tool that is useful in understanding an individual's concept of health and experience with changing behavior.

The Concepts of Health and Wellness

"Health is a state of complete physical, mental and social well-being and not merely the absence of disease or infirmity" (WHO, 2003). Wellness focuses on additional dimensions including the spiritual, emotional, and intellectual elements of well-being. This state is considered to be an "actively sought goal" rather than a chance outcome (Health Promotion Advocates, n.d.). Health and wellness are outcomes that require continual effort to accomplish, rather than a chance happening. This effort

Figure 12-1   Determinants of health.

DETERMINANTS OF HEALTH

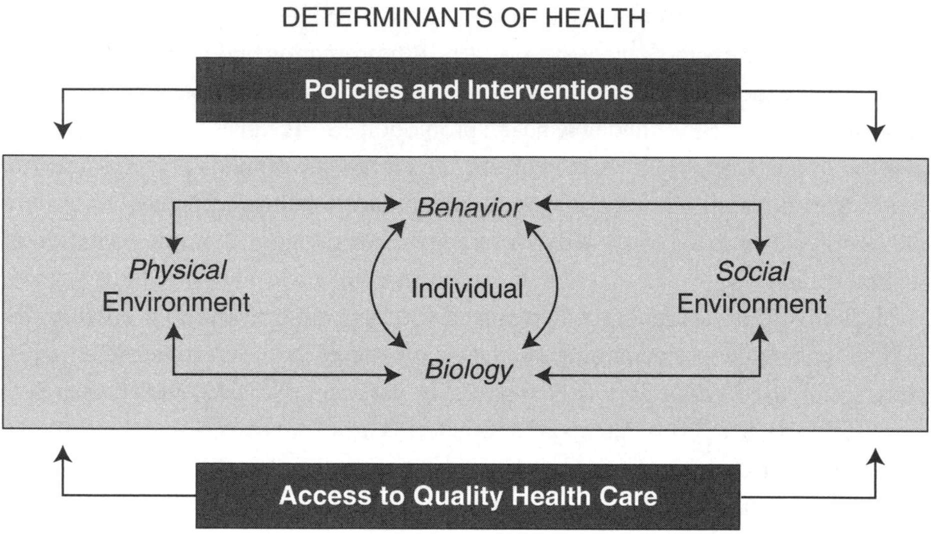

Source: USDHHS, 2000, p. 18.

requires knowledge of healthy behavior, as well as risk of disease, to reach the goal of wellness. Similarly, healthiness also requires effort on the part of the individual. Leddy (2006a) describes a theory of healthiness that considers healthiness as dynamic, goal oriented, and connected to purpose and power.

Figure 12-1 is a view of the *Healthy People 2010* assessment of the determinants of health. According to *Healthy People 2010,* health is determined by a combination of factors including individual behavior and biology, physical and social environment, policy, and access to quality care. Biology is a combination of inborn traits and the effects of life circumstances such as age and habits (diet, drugs, etc.) that can alter the structure and function of the body. Some of these life factors are outside of individual control, age, for example, whereas some are behaviorally influenced. Diet, exercise, and substance use can be within the control of the individual, but influenced by social environment. Physical environment also plays a role in individual health by exposure to toxins and unsafe air, and water and food quality, which have both immediate and long-term effects. The physical environment can be a source of positive health outcomes by encouraging physical activity and significant and safe opportunities to engage in health-promoting behaviors such as sports and fitness (USDHHS, 2000, p. 18).

Access to quality care is also a health determinant. Provision of quality health-care services serves the purpose of diagnosing and treating health problems (secondary and tertiary prevention) and encourages the adoption of healthful habits. This is facilitated by regular opportunities for patients to have education and counseling with skilled providers (primary prevention). Quality care includes providing feedback on progression of health goals, a valuable motivational tool (USDHHS, 2000, p. 18).

The *Healthy People 2010* initiative stresses the impact of individual health on the community; healthy people make health communities. Making our communities and nation models of healthful behavior will ensure healthy living for future generations. This is done through primary, secondary, and tertiary strategies.

Health Promotion and Disease Prevention

Health promotion and disease prevention have gained world attention in recent decades, integral to increasing individual wellness and the health of communities and nations. The CNL attends to prevention rather than merely treatment of disease, projected to have a significant effect on the healthcare economy. The U.S. Surgeon General's reports on the health promotion date back to 1979 (Pender, Murdaugh, & Parsons, 2006, p. 6) and evolve to the *Healthy People* initiatives. This initiative includes surveillance of major indicators of health and use of data to promote achievement of national health goals. The most recent iteration of *Healthy People 2010* includes healthful individual living and the impact of the individuals' health on healthy communities.

Overarching goals of *Healthy People* 2010 are to increase the quality and years of healthy life and to reduce health disparities (USDHHS, n.d.). The first goal challenges the individual to examine lifestyle factors that may reduce the length and quality of the life span. This shifts the focus of the healthcare industry from prevention to cure. *Healthy People 2010* has identified the importance of health lifestyle information and education (USDHHS, n.d.). Unfortunately, this (and other issues such as technology) has resulted in an abundance of available information, not all accurate. The CNL is strategically positioned to partner with patients to develop strategies to initiate and maintain healthier lifestyles focusing on human response to symptoms and diagnoses.

Disease prevention according to Pender is more accurately termed *health protection*. The actual behaviors of health protection may include those of primary,

Box 12-1   Healthy People 2010 Leading Health Indicators

- Physical activity
- Overweight and obesity
- Tobacco use
- Substance abuse
- Responsible sexual behavior
- Mental health
- Injury and violence
- Environmental quality
- Immunization
- Access to health care

Source: USDHHS, n.d.

secondary, and tertiary prevention. Primary prevention activities are those activities that are directed at avoidance of an illness or health problem before it occurs (Clark, 2008, p. 30). Secondary prevention includes measures directed toward early treatment of disease, preventing complications or more serious effects of the illness (Clark, 2008, p. 30). The CNL as the designer, manager, and coordinator of care uses these principles to enhance patients' quality of life and self-management. Tertiary prevention strategies, such as engaging in physical activity to rehabilitate an injury, allow the individual to limit the overall effect of an illness (Clark, 2008, p. 30). The tendency to use the terms *health promotion* and *health protection* interchangeably is easily understandable. However, the outcomes of the behaviors may be truly distinct.

Role of Lifestyle in Disease Prevention

Alterations in lifestyle can and do influence health. In examining the *Healthy People 2010* leading health indicators (USDHHS, n.d.), it is clear that modification of behaviors and lifestyle influences health protection as well as health promotion. In examining the list, 10 of the leading indicators (see Box 12-1) are behavior issues that individuals, families, and community groups (for example, schools) can address to improve health or prevent disease.

The CNL advocates for individuals, families, and communities. For example, making lifestyle changes to increase physical activity and exercise can have a positive influence on prevention of diseases such as coronary artery disease, stroke, diabetes, and multiple other health concerns (USDHHS, n.d.). The influence of exercise in mood can result in reduction of depression and anxiety, improving overall mental as well as physical well-being. Reduction of BMI (body mass index) to a healthy range, as suggested by *Healthy People 2010*, also has a positive influence on overall health and well-being, and it contributes positively to cardiac and diabetes risk reduction (USDHHS, n.d.). Yet, most adults in America do not engage in regular physical activity, and statistics note that adults continue to struggle with weight (http://www.cdc.gov/nchs/fastats/overwt.htm). The CNL engages the head and heart of staff, patients, and families.

Theoretical Models of Behavior Change

Health promotion and disease prevention strategies may require alteration in behavior, or lifestyle changes. Whether considering behavior change to promote health or prevent disease, it is helpful for the CNL to utilize theoretical concepts in planning client care. Two theoretical models of behavior change, the health belief model and Pender's health promotion model, will be discussed here (Pender et al., 2006, p. 38).

The health belief model (HBM) is described as a widely studied and useful theory in understanding factors associated with health behaviors (Daddario, 2007, p. 363). The HBM, originally developed by Becker and Rosenstock et al. in the mid-1960s, examines five major perceptions of clients that determine behavior change to prevent illness: (1) perceived susceptibility, (2) perceived severity, (3) perceived benefits, (4) perceived barriers, and (5) self-efficacy (Daddario, 2007, p. 363). Perceived susceptibility is the individual's own perception of their risk for illness. Self-efficacy, which is integral to the health belief model, is the individual's perception of success.

The second theory of health promotion is Pender's health promotion model (HPM). This model is based on several other behavioral models including the HBM. It identifies numerous factors to the client's success at achieving a change in health-related behaviors. The HPM includes individual's characteristics and behavior conditions that affect the ultimate behavioral outcomes. Much like the health belief model, the HPM looks at perceived benefits, barriers, and self-efficacy as they relate to a proposed change in behavior; however, Pender's model adds the element of *activity-related affect*, or an assessment of how the client feels about changing the behavior. This important element allows for assessment of the client's emotional response toward the change in behavior and anticipated outcome. For example, when counseling a client on weight loss and increasing physical activity to reduce elevated blood pres-

Figure 12-2 Pender's health promotion model (HPM).

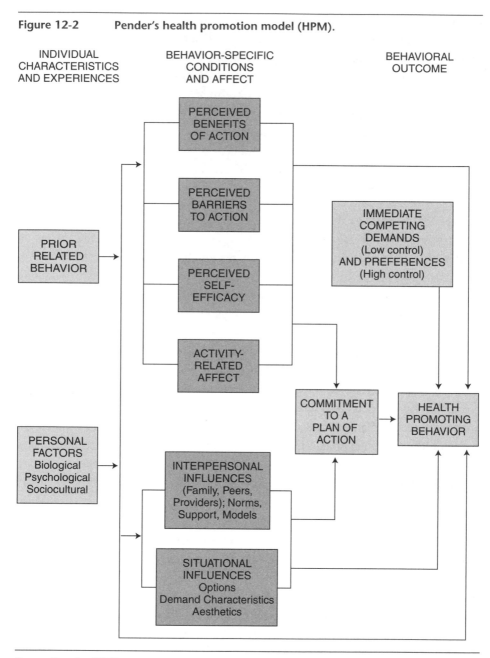

Source: Pender, 2001.

sure, the CNL may make the assumption that everyone would find this an acceptable goal. But the client may have many hidden reasons for not viewing this in a positive light, such as the role that illness may play in the client's life or the social isolation that may be achieved by being inactive or overweight. Addressing the affective result is an important element for successful lifestyle modification that may be overlooked.

Pender's model addresses the interpersonal and situation factors that influence commitment to positive behavior change. The influence of family, friends, and social norms are significant in terms of making lifestyle changes. If there is pressure from the social group or family to continue an unhealthy behavior, the individual may see the benefit of continuing the behavior to be more appealing than the benefit of adopting a healthy alternative. The CNL must be aware of these influences and take them into consideration when developing an action plan with the client.

Once there is a commitment to an action plan, the CNL works with the individual to assist in dealing with competing demands as well as individual needs and preferences. The CNL is an important influence in helping the individual to realize that issues causing setbacks will occur and that behavioral change requires continual effort.

Role of the CNL in Health Promotion and Disease Prevention

The CNL is in a unique position to work with the healthcare team to identify individual needs of clients and families in disease prevention strategies through the lateral integration of care (Begun, Hamilton, Tornabeni, & White, 2006). The main purpose is the achievement of quality outcomes by overseeing and coordinating the work of the team and ensuring that the complexities of client care are addressed. This outcomes-focused role allows the CNL to ensure that the often overlooked (due to lack of time, resources, and appropriately trained staff) area of prevention is addressed. The CNL can take the initial data gathered on admission and utilize it to develop a more comprehensive assessment of this client. The CNL considers the microsystems' processes and patterns related to managing health promotion and disease prevention. The CNL may serve in the capacity of educator, information gatherer, and coordinator to ensure that the client has a plan of health promotion in place. This may include management plans for medications, diet, and other lifestyle modifications to improve patient well-being.

Patient and Family Healthcare Education

Patient education is a role of the CNL supported by professional standards (Bastable, 2008, pp. 4–5). The knowledge and skills needed for appropriate management of a

Box 12-2   Literacy and Preventive Health Behaviors

In a study by White, Chen, and Atchinson published in the *American Journal of Health Behavior* (2008), the relationship between literacy levels and preventive health measures was studied. The National Assessment of Adult Literacy, as well as a background questionnaire, was used to measure health literacy and oral reading fluency.

The study concluded that the relationship between health literacy and preventive health behaviors varies by age. In adults between 16 and 64 years, there was no relationship between health literacy level and self-report of most preventive health behaviors. In those over age 65, the relationship between health literacy and report of preventive health measures was positive. The preventive health behaviors evaluated in this study included mammography, dental care, vision care, colon screening, osteoporosis screening, prostate screening, and flu and pneumonia vaccinations.

The clinical nurse leader may find this study useful as a basis for planning health promotion activities and materials, but also to develop further research regarding motivation of individuals to participate in or avoid preventive health measures.

Source: White, Chen, & Atchinson, 2008.

client at home may actually come from multiple sources, making the risk of confusion high. For example, the CNL provides the client with written information and verbal explanations of medications and treatments required at home. The respiratory therapist may be the one to teach the client about use of an inhaler, and the nutritionist may be responsible for teaching the dietary portion of the treatment plan. Any slight variation in the instructions can cause confusion for the client and family, resulting in serious errors or omissions in care. This makes the CNL, as lateral integrator of care, crucial to achieving quality client outcomes through education. The CNL will need input from multiple members of the team to ensure continuity and compliance. The CNL ensures that instruction plans and materials are consistent across disciplines, appropriate to the patient population, and individualized to meet patient and family needs and schedules. This, in short, makes the role of the CNL in health education multilayered.

The CNL may be responsible for the identification or development of materials that are appropriately individualized to patient and family needs. The CNL may also serve as a support person for staff-level primary nurses in the delivery of a comprehensive patient education plan, or he or she may take the responsibility of delivering the education.

Issue of Health Literacy in Health Education

Literacy in general remains a concern in the United States, with an estimated 14% of the adult population demonstrating literacy below what is considered a basic level (ProLiteracy, 2006). Individuals in this reading category may be unable to complete simple tasks or follow basic directions. Further information indicates that "a third of American adults—some 89 million people—lack sufficient health literacy to effectively undertake and execute needed medical treatments and preventative health care" (Weiss, 2007, p. 7). This problem costs billions of dollars per year.

Health literacy is not simply the ability to read health information but encompasses the client's ability to interpret instructions, read medication labels, and follow directions on medical technology items utilized in care management. Patients and their family caregivers are bombarded with health and wellness information from numerous sources that must be sifted through in order to judge its accuracy and applicability. Murphy-Knoll (2007) describes the problem of low health literacy as "so common in America that it puts at risk countless numbers of patients who cannot comprehend the information required to seek or receive quality healthcare." (p. 207). The Joint Commission has identified the patient's right to receive information in a way understandable to them. Lack of this essential level of communication is a patent safety concern, as confirmed by Joint Commission data, which identifies that "65% of errors reported involve communication breakdown" (Murphy-Knoll, 2007, p. 208). Further, health literacy is identified in *Healthy People 2010* as a vital element in achievement of national health goals (USDHHS, 2000).

The availability of information to the consumer has made the job of the healthcare professional more of a challenge. The CNL needs to be well read and current on not only the legitimate health information but also the less accurate information to ensure that the client receives the best information possible. The CNL may also need to teach patients and families how to evaluate journals, books, and Internet sources to determine their validity as reliable sources of health information.

The CNL can play an essential role in assessment of the patient's ability to read and understand education material. Although a patient's level of formal education is

Figure 12-3   Example of simple signange.

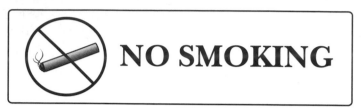

not an indicator of reading and comprehension ability, it is useful information in a larger picture of health literacy. Matching material to the patient's reading and comprehension level may increase the patient's ability to follow complicated management regimens.

Patient education material or instructions that the patient and family may need to carry out self-care activities in the home can be evaluated by using one of many tools available to measure the grade level of the piece. SMOG (simple measure of gobbledygook) is one of the assessment tools considered to be reliable and valid in its ability to predict grade level of written material. This evaluation is performed by counting the number of multisyllable words in a passage, and it will determine grade level as low as grade 4 (Bastable, 2008, p. 184).

In addition to determining the grade level of material used in patient and family education and discharge materials, the CNL can employ other strategies within the healthcare institution to further address the issue of health literacy. Working with ancillary departments to make the institution friendly to those with low literacy or limited English language skills by using simple, clear signage that employs figures and easily recognizable symbols such as that in Figure 12-3 ensures that all who enter the facility have an opportunity for a safe, effective stay.

The CNL is integral to promoting institutional policy regarding the identification of patients with low literacy levels. Additionally, the CNL can be instrumental in developing relationships with community programs to assist with strategies for ensuring safe communications while the patient is in the institution. The CNL can use referral sources for postdischarge improvement of health literacy skills. The CNL is responsible for raising the awareness of the nursing staff of the issue of health literacy and encouraging documentation of reading and communication issues that can impact client care. Instructing staff on simple measures of determining the grade level of common materials such as consents, instructions sheets, and direc-

Box 12-3 Using the SMOG Method

Apply the SMOG method to the simplified directions below.

Directions for Wet-to-Dry Sterile Dressing Change

Use a clean, dry surface for the procedure. Gather all equipment for the dressing change. Open all packages, being careful to avoid touching the new dressing. Remove old dressing using clean gloves, and discard into a trash can. Wet sterile gauze pads with sterile saline. Apply clean gloves. Cleanse the wound with the moist gauze pads. Start at the center, and move out to the edge of the wound. Apply moist gauze pads to cover the wound. Cover the moist pads with dry gauze pads. Tape the new dressing in place. Discard all used equipment.

1. There are 5 polysyllabic words.
2. There are 13 sentences.
3. There are 0.4 polysyllabic words per sentence.
4. $0.4 \times 13 = 5.2$
5. $5.2 + 5 = 10.2$
6. 9 is the nearest perfect square. 3 is the square root. 3 + 3 (constant) = 6
This piece has a grade level of 6.

Source: Harvard School of Public Health, 2005.

tions on emergency care, and rewriting these materials to meet the needs of the patient, is an easy method of addressing this safety concern.

In developing patient education materials or writing discharge instructions, replacing medical terms with common, everyday language can greatly reduce the reading level while increasing the patient's ability to understand instructions. For example, replacing terms such as *hypertension* with *high blood pressure*, or *menstruation* with *period* can help the patient understand and more closely follow directions for care (Weiss, 2007, p. 33). The CNL may also opt to adapt commonly used materials to a nonwritten format such as video or DVD to enhance patient comprehension (Weiss, 2007, p. 43).

Other assessment data that the CNL may need is information about any physical impairment that may affect the patient's ability to comprehend health information. Specifically, vision and hearing impairments may impact the patient's ability to read the written word or to hear the spoken word. These issues may be a source of embarrassment to the patient, who may not report these problems readily and leave the situation unprepared to participate in self-care. Alternative methods of delivering essential information may need to be developed to ensure that the patient has the needed information. These disabilities are education issues, and may affect management of diseases as well. For example, a patient may need precise doses of a medication but may be unable to see the medication vial or read the pill bottle. Assessment and addressing this issue is important to the education plan for the patient.

Low health literacy has an affect on the economy as well. The complexities of technology and dependency on written instructions in high-level English puts those with low literacy, the elderly, and those with chronic conditions at risk of errors in care due to misunderstanding. This population is at greater risk of readmission to healthcare facilities because of these issues, leading to increased healthcare costs, likely higher than for the average population (Pawlak, 2005, p. 173). The efforts of the CNL to bridge this gap can have a direct impact on cost reduction and improving care, making the business case for change.

Role of the CNL in Assessment, Planning, Implementing, and Evaluating Healthcare Education

The CNL plays a vital role in the assessing, planning, implementing, and evaluating the education needs of clients and families. The lateral integration role of the CNL is critical to ensuring that the education needs are met. CNL are generalists, enabling them to move between patient populations based on disease category and to carry out many nursing roles to achieve high-quality client care.

Culturally Competent Healthcare Management

The term *cultural competence* has become a buzzword in health care and healthcare education. This term can also have many definitions with slight variations. For the purposes of this discussion, we will use the following definition, put forth by transcultural nursing (culturaldiversity.org, 1997–2008b): "Cultural competence is obtaining cultural information and then applying that knowledge. This cultural awareness allows you to see the entire picture and improves the quality of care and health outcomes." Transcultural nursing considers that organizations are culturally competent when they create an atmosphere that values differences and is aware of culture as evidenced by assessment and recognition of situations that arise when cultures interact. This is manifested by an institution that has knowledge of its own culture and adapts policy and service delivery to be open to all levels of diversity (cultural-diversity.org, 1997–2008b). It is apparent from this comprehensive definition that cultural diversity is far more encompassing than simply asking a patient about food preferences, religious practices, or country of birth. Culture is a learned set of behaviors and a way of thinking that guides life. It includes social norms and life practices (culturaldiversity.org, 1997–2008a).

Although race and ethnicity can play a role in culture, culture extends beyond these factors. For example, gay and lesbian individuals have learned behaviors and norms that connect them as a cultural group. Care for gay and lesbian patients requires not only knowledge of the needs of the individual patient, but the norms of the cultural as interpreted by the client, and awareness on the provider's part regarding his or her thoughts and feelings about this particular cultural group.

To be culturally competent healthcare providers and to function as integrators of care, CNLs must be self-aware of feelings and prejudices about what is considered "right" or "acceptable." It is a professional responsibility to be aware of the world around them to gain an understanding of various groups and their healthcare values and practices. This self-awareness and commitment to enhanced cultural knowledge translates into development of culturally appropriate plans of care and encourages healthcare organizations to promote culturally diverse policy and practice (Leddy, 2006b, p. 174–176).

The CNL can serve as an ambassador to ensure that culturally sensitive practices are given appropriate levels of priority when delivering care to the diverse population. This should begin by reviewing how a patient moves through the organization and identifying where elements of culture may be ignored or lack integration. Review the process of admission, for example. Are there methods of assessing the cultural practices that can be integrated into care? Is information gathered about religious or spiritual practices, diet, daily routine and activity, and alternative health practices so that these can be built into daily care routines? These are simple changes that highlight the importance of diversity and cultural practices into the provision of quality care.

Food plays a variety of roles in many cultural groups. Many view food as having healing properties. In encouraging the wife of an elderly man at the end of life to continue to bring home-cooked food to the patient, the CNL is recognizing the value of food in not only the couple's culture, but in their relationship as well.

There are many examples of healthcare providers ignoring a patient's culture and imposing the norms of the organization or the individual provider on the patient. A lesbian woman may be offended when the nurse who admits her persists in using the term *homosexual* rather than the often preferred term *lesbian* and not gathering information regarding the woman's partner, but rather asking for contact information for her parents. The use of the term *homosexual* can be offensive to some gay and lesbian individuals. Recognition should be given to the same-sex partner as being an important and significant person.

As a further example, a technician working with an elderly female client is over-heard to call the patient "honey" or by her first name. After the technician leaves, the CNL overhears the patient tell her roommate, "I keep telling them that I am Mrs. Johnson, but they keep calling me honey." Use of a proper name and title is a show of respect and recognition of worth. Overfamiliarity is felt to be demeaning and dis-respectful. All of the above situations give examples of lack of awareness of cultural diversity that can be a barrier to effective care.

In terms of health promotion, culture becomes paramount. Health promotion and disease prevention must consider the individual patient's cultural norms to be suc-cessful. Lifestyle is in fact a part of culture. Encouraging regular visits to the primary care provider may not be accepted by an individual whose culture dictates that doc-tors are only consulted during acute illness, or not at all. Teaching preventive care practices may not be readily acceptable by members of a cultural group who believe in ancient alternative methods of care. These practices can in some cases be incor-porated into plans of health promotion.

Culture can extend to the American workforce as a cultural group as well. Many people in the corporate workforce work long hours, eat poorly, and engage in little exercise. This is promoted by the corporate culture. The CNL needs to take lifestyle factors into account when working with these clients to recognize heath issues and incorporate healthful habits into their high-pressure lives.

The role of the CNL in managing care from a culturally competent perspective is supported by the work of Dr. Madeleine Leininger; Dr. Leininger developed the theory of cultural care diversity and universality to improve nursing care through recognition of the significant impact of culture on health, illness, and dying practices. Leininger's theory supports the role of nursing as "essentially a transcultural care pro-fession and discipline" that is the means by which culturally competent care can be delivered (Parker, 2006, p. 315). The CNL should lead the way in knowledge of the influence of culture as well as the integration of cultural influences throughout the patient care experience. This is manifested through the CNL's role in direct patient care, manager of care, and educator.

The CNL is positioned to be a force in nursing care in the 21st century because of the generalist focus, providing a broad basis of knowledge and experience to the care of patients. This is made more important by the attention that the CNL can give to the health issues facing the population in the future. This future focus allows the CNL to assist patients and families to maintain optimum health through counseling and education to modify lifestyle and risk. Recognition of literacy and cultural factors that often go overlooked in high-acuity health care can be addressed by the clinical nurse leader.

Tools of the Trade: Case Studies

Case Study 1: Ms. M., Part 1

Let's apply the concepts discussed throughout the chapter to the case of Ms. M., a 64-year-old patient admitted to the hospital from her primary care provider's office. The admitting diagnosis is acute pylonephritis. The admission history reveals that Ms. M. has had recurrent urinary tract infections over the course of the last year that were treated with oral antimicrobials. Ms. M. has a BMI of 31 and is not physically active. Laboratory results show fasting blood glucose of 310 mg/dl and a hemoglobin A1C (glycoselated hemoglobin) of 8.2. Ms. M. is told by her provider that she has diabetes and will need to learn to manage her condition at home.

The CNL reviews the chart and consults with the staff nurse caring for Ms. M. in order to begin to assess the needs of the client. The R.N. reports that Ms. M. is a pleasant but anxious patient. She was very emotional about the diagnosis of diabetes and told the nurse that her mother and grandmother were both diabetic and suffered serious complications of the disease such as blindness and "sores" that never healed. On admission Ms. M. reported that she left high school before graduating to get married. She recently earned her GED, which was a lifelong goal. The CNL finds that Ms. M. has reported that she has not felt well for "a long time" and is discouraged by the weight gain over the past several years, lack of energy for physical activity, and loss of interest in gardening and crafts, which she previously enjoyed. When the CNL meets Ms. M. in her room, the patient tells the CNL that she is extremely upset by the hospitalization and diabetes diagnosis and that she had always been a "very healthy" person.

1. Is Ms. M. a healthy person?
2. What role can the CNL play in this case with the information currently available?
3. What primary, secondary, and tertiary prevention strategies can be employed?

Case Study 1: Ms. M., Part 2

Returning to the case of Ms. M., the CNL notes that her BMI on admission was 31, which falls in the obese range. Although the available diagnostic data do not reveal evidence of cardiovascular disease, the diagnosis of diabetes, lack of physical activity, and progressive weight gain do put Ms. M. at an increased risk for development of cardiovascular disease. The CNL determines that a more complete assessment of lifestyle factors, including dietary patterns, alcohol and tobacco use, and actual physical ability, should be completed before developing a complete plan of care for Ms. M.

During interview with Ms. M., the CNL learns that this patient consumes most of her daily calories from refined starches and high-fat animal products. She mentions that since the children have left the home, she and her husband "can't be bothered" to cook and often order takeout for meals. She adds that the weight gain makes no sense to her because she generally eats only one meal a day, at the dinner hour. During the daytime hours she drinks coffee and tea and occasionally makes a sandwich with cheese and bread. Both Mr. and Ms. M. mention that they used to love the vegetables from their home garden, but neither has interest in maintaining a garden any longer. Ms. M. shares that she smoked in high school, but quit when she was pregnant with the first of her three pregnancies. She began smoking again about 10 years ago and is currently smoking almost a pack a day. In the last year or so, she has developed "trouble sleeping" that she attributed to nerves and caffeine intake. She has tried to cut out coffee in the late afternoon and evening hours, but finds that she still does not sleep well. She does not use prescription sleeping pills, but does take over-the-counter sleeping aids about one to two times per week.

1. Using the information gathered thus far, what risk factors should the CNL address in a plan?
2. What other information is needed in order to develop a comprehensive plan based in theory?

Case Study 1: Ms. M., Part 3

Ms. M. further reinforces her anger and frustration as a newly diagnosed diabetic to the CNL. She has had several family members with this disease, and they had complications that were "awful." She does not want to live like that. She also shares that she remembers her mother never being able to eat "normal" food and taking shots of insulin. When the topic of cardiovascular risk is mentioned, Ms. M. states that there is no heart disease in her family, so she never really worried about it. She is not aware that diabetes increases her risk for cardiac disease. She is concerned that her smoking history increases her cancer risk and has thought about quitting. The CNL questions Ms. M. about past attempts at changing behaviors. Ms. M. tells the nurse that she had no trouble quitting smoking, but that was years ago and she was motivated by her pregnancies. She would like to be more active again, but doesn't really know how to start. She also freely admits a fear of failure.

1. How does this information assist the CNL? What other information is needed?
2. What information should the CNL be sure is included in a teaching plan before Ms. M. is discharged? What information is important but not a priority at this time?
3. How would the CNL link Ms. M. to community resources? How does Ms. M.'s history or her past lifestyle guide this discussion?

Summary

- Many of the healthcare issues facing Americans are preventable and can be addressed through alterations in lifestyle and environment.
- As hospital stays shorten, the ability of nurses to address issues, such as the lifestyle factors that may contribute to disease risk, is drastically reduced. The CNL is integral in prioritizing need and planning care to address these concerns.
- Access to quality care encourages the adoption of healthful habits by giving the patient regular opportunities for education and counseling with skilled providers such as a CNL.
- Health literacy is a growing concern regarding the ability of the individual to comprehend health instructions.
- It is the responsibility of CNLs to be aware of the world around them to gain an understanding of various cultural groups and their healthcare values and practices.

Reflection Questions

1. Differentiate health promotion from disease prevention. Give an example of each.
2. Select one of the health indicators from *Healthy People 2010*. Discuss how alteration in lifestyle can influence this indicator. Give specific examples.
3. How does public policy influence personal health? Give specific examples.
4. Discuss how the CNL can enhance the health literacy of the patient population served.
5. Differentiate between health and wellness.
7. Select a nursing theory, and discuss how this theory applies to health promotion and disease prevention.
8. How can patient and family education be used as a health promotion strategy? How does it contribute to disease prevention?
9. Describe culture competence. Differentiate culture from ethnicity.
10. What influence does culture have on health promotion and disease prevention?
11. Describe the role of the CNL in health promotion.

Learning Activities

1. Interview a classmate to identify one to two lifestyle factors that your classmate could modify to improve health status or reduce disease risk. Ask your partner what lifestyle factors are of most concern. Are these the same as the factors that you identified?
2. Develop a plan of health promotion for your partner using the information gathered.

Recommended Reading

Bettcher, D. W. (2007, May 25). Exposure to secondhand smoke among students aged 13–15 years—worldwide, 2000–2007. *Morbidity and Mortality Weekly Report, 56*(20), 497–500.

Blaise, K. K., Hayes, J. S., Kozier, B., & Erb, G. (2006). *Professional nursing practice: Concepts and perspectives* (5th ed.). Upper Saddle River, NJ: Pearson.

Health Promotion Advocates. (n.d.). *Definitions*. Retrieved June 9, 2008, from http://healthpromotionadvocates.org/resources/definitions.htm

McCarthy, C. (2007, September 17). Raising healthy kids: A Harvard pediatrician replies to parents worried about day care, autism and vaccines. *Newsweek, 150*(12). Retrieved May 14, 2009, from http://www.newsweek.com/id/40753

World Health Organization (WHO). (2003). *WHO definition of health*. Retrieved June 9, 2008, from http://www.who.int/about/definition/en/print.html

References

American Association of Colleges of Nursing (AACN). (2003). *White paper on the role of the clinical nurse leader.* Retrieved June 12, 2008, from http://www.aacn.nche.edu/ publications/whitepapers/ClinicalNurseLeader.htm

Bastable, S. B. (2008). *Essentials of patient education.* Sudbury, MA: Jones and Bartlett.

Begun, J. W., Hamilton, J. A., Tornabeni, J., & White, K. R. (2006). Opportunities for improving patient care through lateral integration: The clinical nurse leader. *Journal of Healthcare Management, 51*(1), 19–25.

Clark, M. J. (2008). *Community health nursing: Advocacy for population health* (5th ed.). Upper Saddle River, NJ: Pearson.

culturaldiversity.org. (1997–2008a). *The basic concepts of transcultural nursing.* Retrieved June 9, 2008, from http://www.culturediversity.org/basic.htm

culturaldiversity.org. (1997–2008b). *Cultural competence.* Retrieved June 8, 2008, from http://www.culturediversity.org/cultcomp.htm

Daddario, D. K. (2007). *A review of the use of the health belief model for weight management. MED-SURG Nursing, 16*(6), 363–366.

Harvard School of Public Health/Department of Society, Human Development, and Health. (2005). *Health literacy: How to test for readability.* Retrieved June 6, 2008, from http://www.hsph.harvard.edu/healthliteracy/how_to/smog_2.pdf

Leddy, S. K. (2006a). *Health promotion: Mobilizing strengths to enhance health, wellness and well-being.* Sudbury, MA: Jones and Bartlett.

Leddy, S. K. (2006b). *Integrative health promotion: Conceptual basis for nursing practice* (2nd ed.). Sudbury, MA: Jones and Bartlett.

Murphy-Knoll, L. (2007). Low health literacy puts patients at risk: The Joint Commission proposes solutions to a national problem. *Journal of Nursing Care Quality, 22*(3), 205–209.

National Center for Health Statistics. (2007). *Health, United States 2007, with chartbook on trends in the health of Americans.* Hyattsville, MD: Author.

Parker, M. E. (2006). *Nursing theories and nursing practice* (2nd ed). Philadelphia: F. A. Davis.

Pawlak, R. (2005). Economic considerations of health literacy. *Nursing Economics, 23*(4), 173–180.

Pender, N. J. (2001). *Health promotion model* (revised). Retrieved June 6, 2008, from http://www.nursing.umich.edu/faculty/pender/chart.gif

Pender, N. J., Murdaugh, C. L., & Parsons, M. A. (2006). *Health promotion in nursing practice* (5th ed.). Upper Saddle River, NJ: Pearson.

ProLiteracy Worldwide. (2006). *The state of adult literacy 2006.* Retrieved April 1, 2009, from http://www.proliteracy.org/NetCommunity/Document.Doc?id=14

U.S. Department of Health and Human Services (USDHHS). (2000). *Healthy People 2010: Understanding and improving health* (2nd ed.). Washington, DC: U.S. Government Printing Office.

U.S. Department of Health and Human Services (USDHHS). (n.d.). *Healthy People 2010.* Retrieved June 9, 2008, from http://www.healthypeople.gov

Weiss, B. D. (2007). *Health literacy and patient safety: Help patients understand; Manual for clinicians* (2nd ed). Chicago: American Medical Association Foundation.

White, S, Chen, J., & Atchinson, R. (2008). Relationship of preventative health practices and literacy: A national study. *American Journal of Health Behavior, 32*(3), 227–242.

Unit 6

Academic and Clinical Foundations for Successful CNL Matriculation

THIRTEEN

Curriculum Issues for CNL Academic Programs

■ Debra C. Davis and Catherine Dearman

■ **Learning Objectives**

■ Discuss the didactic content and curriculum issues in developing CNLs.
■ Differentiate academic content and clinical experiences for various entries for the CNL.
■ Examine curricular models for educating CNLs.

"If our work, at its core, is 'to heal and help' people in distress, then we can get great benefit and guidance for our actions by seeing the work and then figuring out how we can best help that."

Donald Berwick

Key Terms

Advanced nurse generalist

Clinical microsystems

CNL Roles

Clinician

Client advocate

Manager   ·

Lifelong learner

Systems analyst/risk anticipator

Outcomes manager

Team educator

Member of a profession

Information manager

CNL Professional Values

Altruism

Human dignity

Social justice

Accountability

Integrity

CNL Core Competencies

Critical thinking

Ethics

Human diversity

Member of a profession

Health promotion, risk reduction,
   and disease prevention

Information and healthcare
   technologies

Designer/manager/coordinator
   of comprehensive care

Communication

Assessment

Global health care

Nursing technology and resource
   management

Illness and disease management

Healthcare systems and policy knowledge

Provider and manager of care

Introduction

The educational preparation of the clinical nurse leader (CNL) offers many curricular challenges and may or may not fit the mold of other master's programs in nursing. The CNL is a new and evolving role and, as such, creates some faculty concerns that become opportunities when designing curricula for educating CNL students. Opportunities include, first and foremost, that educators more than likely were not educated as a CNL. Designing curricula to prepare CNLs when not prepared in that specific area may be an issue when the role is not universally adopted in healthcare organizations. Enthusiasm for the role and the anticipated impact that it will have on the future of health care must be translated into discrete courses for students. Faculty are further challenged when designing clinical learning opportunities for students when few or no practicing CNLs are available to serve as preceptors and mentors for students. Therefore, faculty developing CNL programs will be tasked not only with designing the curriculum but also with marketing the role to clinical partners, educating the staff in those facilities, and recruiting students who have not considered the role.

Educating and Socializing the CNL

The CNL graduate cannot know everything involved in producing a safe, high-quality, cost-effective patient care environment, but faculty must ensure curricula that allow each participant to learn the essential skills. Quality, safety, and evidence-based practice issues are cornerstones for preparation of the CNL. The fragmentation of care and increase in errors affecting the health of patients in our current health system are well documented in the literature. Clinical nurse leaders, advanced generalists who practice at the point of care, are a key variable in designing an effective solution to the quality care issues so prevalent in health care today. The CNL graduate is prepared to direct, coordinate, and evaluate patient care at the microsystems' level in a variety of healthcare settings, including community. The effectiveness of the CNL is dependent on a clear understanding of construction and function of microsystems, the facilitation and performance of teams, and the incorporation of the best research and best practices into all levels of care to improve patient safety, health outcomes, and the effective organization of systems. Leadership development is a critical element in each of the factors above. CNL students must be prepared to serve as leaders and innovators for all nursing staff. Educational efforts and the process of socializing CNLs into the profession must build on and, as appropriate, modify values and behavior patterns developed early in life. Values are difficult to teach as part of professional education. Nevertheless, CNL faculty must design learning opportunities that support empathic, sensitive, and compassionate care for individuals, groups, and communities; that promote and reward honesty and accountability; that make students aware of social and ethical issues; and that nurture students' awareness of their own value systems, as well as those of others.

As CNL students and graduates oversee the care coordination of a distinct group of patients and provide direct care in complex situations, putting evidence-based practice into action can ensure that patients benefit from the latest innovations in care delivery. The curriculum will provide opportunities to develop cultural competency and competencies in leadership, evaluating patient outcomes, assessing cohort risks, and perfecting decision-making skills. This will serve to improve the quality of patient care and educate nurses who are better prepared to thrive in the healthcare system. Designing curricula to address such a diverse array of roles and competencies presents an exquisite opportunity for nurse educators, who for many years have focused their attention on preparing specialists. Nurse educators are charged to create curricula that are flexible, offer multiple entry and exit points, and address the most acute issues in nursing today: well-prepared nurses who can assume leadership roles in a complex and fragmented healthcare system to bring order out of chaos.

Although specific courses and curricula will vary, CNL education must include a strong base in the physical and social sciences as well as learning experiences in philosophy, the arts, and humanities. Recent and evolving trends in health care require particular emphasis on learning related to economics, environmental science, epidemiology, genetics, gerontology, global perspectives, informatics, organizations and systems, and communications. The successful integration of liberal education and professional education requires guidance from faculty to help students build bridges between general concepts and practice. Making these connections enables students to use what they have learned to understand situations in nursing practice. Students must be accountable for previous knowledge just as faculty are responsible for building on that foundation, facilitating cognitive skill development, and encouraging lifelong learning. Professional education must build upon the competencies, knowledge, and skills acquired through liberal education courses.

CNL Curricular Options for Schools of Nursing

Educational preparation for the CNL occurs at the master's level and builds on a liberal education foundation and the competencies for the baccalaureate in nursing. In developing the curriculum, faculty have a variety of resources at their disposal, including *The Essentials of Master's Education for Advanced Practice Nursing* (AACN, 1996) and AACN's *White Paper on the Education and Role of the Clinical Nurse Leader* (2007). These documents identify essential content and clinical experiences and outline core competencies for the CNL. How a faculty group organizes these requirements into specific courses will vary, influenced by the mission of the school, school policies for graduate programs, specific characteristics of the student population, and needs of the clinical partners. All programs must prepare students to sit for certification, and therefore students are expected to have at least 500 clinical hours including a clinical immersion experience in the CNL role. The majority of graduate programs offer part-time study for the CNL, and many offer courses fully online. These options allow students to continue to work while earning their MSN degree. High-quality courses for the CNL can be offered fully online. Faculty development and support is important in designing, implementing, evaluating, and maintaining academic integrity of these courses, just as with courses offered on campus.

CNL Curricular Models

A variety of curricular models have been developed by schools of nursing for the CNL role. The following section presents curricular options for a CNL program. Course titles, program objectives, and descriptions from university/college Web sites with CNL programs are provided as examples. These examples, along with a further breakdown of one school's course descriptions to include course objectives, course and clinical assignments, and evaluation methods, will assist faculty in schools to create their own CNL program.

Traditional Post-BSN Preparation

New MSN Programs
Some nursing programs offering advanced generalist (CNL) preparation for students have traditionally offered a BSN only. The national focus on improving quality and safety has sparked interest in the CNL option, and many of these programs have expanded course offerings to prepare CNLs. For these programs, the advanced generalist course work is designed to be completely focused on the CNL. In this case, all core and support courses are based on the CNL competencies and are specifically designed to further the role. For example, if the entire MSN program is focused on preparing CNLs, an evidence-based practice course can develop students' skill sets

with regard to the evidence supporting microsystem issues. Publications focused on improving quality and safety in patient care can be integrated into course work and emphasis can be placed on interprofessional collaboration, all fundamental skills for the clinical nurse leader. One can readily see that such a focused curriculum can achieve an integrated solution to issues and concerns related to patient care, including the following: (a) clinical knowledge, depth, and expertise; (b) critical thinking and problem solving; (c) the need for a strong nursing player on the interdisciplinary team; and (d) a method of integrating evidence-based practice at the patient-provider interface (Bower, 2006). The CNL-focused curriculum can offer students the opportunity to consider all components of health and a healthy work environment, identify point-of-care problems, develop action plans to solve these problems, implement evidence-based interventions in the form of patient care and education, and evaluate the resolution of these problems. The curriculum can then provide opportunities for CNLs to develop cultural competencies and competencies in leadership, evaluating patient outcomes, assessing cohort risks, and perfecting decision-making skills, thereby improving the quality of patient care and educating nurses who are better prepared to thrive in a complex healthcare system.

Most models designed for the registered nurse with a baccalaureate degree in nursing range from 32 to 40 semester credits and require one year of full-time study. Several schools also offer entry-level CNL programs for nonnursing college graduates. These programs typically use an accelerated model for the achievement of baccalaureate nursing competencies and then add on or integrate CNL competencies. Average length of time to complete an entry-level CNL program for nonnursing college graduates is 22 to 24 months. A challenge for faculty in these accelerated models directly related to preparation of CNL competencies is the short time frame for the course of study. Leadership, a critical element of CNL preparation, is a skill set that requires time to build and be integrated into personal practice. Accelerated graduates may not be confident in their leadership capabilities because they question their personal competency in basic nursing skills. The rapid pace of accelerated programs, so prized by programs and faculty alike, may actually be a detriment to the development of leadership qualities.

Registered nurse (RN) to MSN programs are also offered by a number of schools. These programs, designed for associate degree and diploma nurses, facilitate attainment of the MSN degree without having to first obtain a BSN. As with the entry-level option described above, these programs include courses and clinical requirements to ensure that the nurse with an associate degree or diploma achieves baccalaureate nursing competencies and CNL competencies. These programs average 24 months for full-time study.

Expansion of Existing MSN Programs

For schools with existing graduate programs, especially those preparing advance practice nurses, offering an advanced generalist option will require a shift in focus for faculty. A curriculum that has, at its core, the preparation of specialists may not provide the best preparation of an advanced generalist. At a minimum, the faculty will need to address some significant curricular issues. For example, the faculty group will need to decide which, if any, of the existing core courses (typically courses such as Theories in Nursing, Nursing Research/Evidence-Based Practice, and Health Policy) for students in the specialty areas are appropriate for CNL students. For example, is an existing course Health Policy for Advance Practice Nurses (APNs) appropriate for all students? Is there specific content that applies only to APNs or, conversely, to CNLs? Should CNL students be placed in separate sections of such courses or mixed with advanced practice nurses? Can/should the course be modified to meet CNL student needs? If the course is broad enough to address the concerns of CNLs as well as APNs, should the two groups be blended in sections or separated into like sections? If there is a finance course for nurse administrators, is this course appropriate for the CNL? Although the ability to "share" existing core courses with courses needed for the CNL increases efficiency in planning the new curriculum, faculty will need to carefully review existing courses to assure a match with CNL core competencies as well as advance practice competencies.

Schools will also need to determine whether multiple entry points will be offered. Is the program designed just for the post-BSN graduate, or will the program have a track for nurses without a BSN degree, or will it accommodate nurses with other advanced nursing degrees who want to retool as a CNL? Accelerated programs are growing in number and popularity nationwide. Can accelerated graduates be successful in a clinical leadership position? Will they garner the respect they need to be effective in the role?

Academic and Clinical Preparation of CNLs

The academic preparation of the CNL differs from that of a traditional BSN graduate in that the CNL is expected to demonstrate advanced leadership skills to design, coordinate, and evaluate care with increasingly complex and diverse populations in

Figure 13-1 Needs assessment.

The needs assessment assignment provides the background for problem identification to support your particular project. Using a project management methodology and microsystem, consider problem(s) that need to be addressed. Defining the problem and the need to seek solutions is a critical component of project plan. What, as precisely as it can be stated, is the problem? Why is it a problem? For whom is it a problem? Be as concise and clear as possible. Before one can outline project strategies, a clear, concise problem statement (based on needs) will be necessary.

Using a project planning methodology, Lewis (2005) delineated closed-ended and open-ended problems. Closed-ended problems tend to have single solutions; open-ended problems have multiple solutions. Lewis, in support of the importance of constructing a good problem statement, promotes the inclusion of the following items: (1) a clear reflection of shared values and a clear purpose; (2) omitting causes or remedies in the statement itself; (3) defining the problem as manageable processes; (4) including measurable characteristics; and (5) refining the statement as evidence (knowledge) is gained.

Potential alternative solutions need to be outlined as well to form the basis for your project. Your project will address one, or potentially more than one, of the alternatives detailed here. You need to consider the pros and cons of each alternative and consider how your selected alternative (your project) will address the need.

multiple environments. The preparation of the CNL also differs from advanced practice nursing preparation in that the CNL is an advanced generalist and does not specialize. The CNL works in collaboration with advanced practice nurses. Examples of the differentiation between advanced generalists and specialists are provided by AACN in the CNL/CNS comparison paper (2004).

Concepts and content that are important to include in the curriculum to build the CNL clinician role include how to search for research-based clinical guidelines and best practices that will provide opportunities to improve clinical care. Practice guidelines are built on evidence; the CNL must be relentless in demanding that evidence be provided to support every aspect of patient care. The CNL must be skilled in the acquisition and dissemination of knowledge, working in groups, and managing change. In addition to justifying clinical actions based on evidence, the CNL must have the oppor-

Figure 13-2 Outcomes management project.

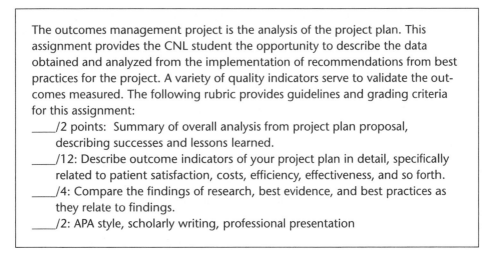

The outcomes management project is the analysis of the project plan. This assignment provides the CNL student the opportunity to describe the data obtained and analyzed from the implementation of recommendations from best practices for the project. A variety of quality indicators serve to validate the outcomes measured. The following rubric provides guidelines and grading criteria for this assignment:

____/2 points: Summary of overall analysis from project plan proposal, describing successes and lessons learned.

____/12: Describe outcome indicators of your project plan in detail, specifically related to patient satisfaction, costs, efficiency, effectiveness, and so forth.

____/4: Compare the findings of research, best evidence, and best practices as they relate to findings.

____/2: APA style, scholarly writing, professional presentation

tunity to locate and apply evidence that challenges current practices/procedures and to incorporate new evidence into practice environments. Practical experience opportunities such as grand rounds, case presentations, and journal clubs may be included in the preparation of CNLs to ensure that new evidence is embedded in clinical practice.

Quality improvement strategies can be the focus of classroom assignments to give students the opportunity to practice communication techniques, role-play processes, and predict outcomes. For example, the five Ps of a clinical microsystem—purpose, patients, professionals, processes, and patterns—can be used with case studies depicting clinical situations to give CNLs the opportunity to practice assessing an environment and proposing solutions to be tested. One way to accomplish the student's true integration of the five Ps can be a needs assessment.

The CNL student also needs to develop competencies in lateral integration of care, microsystem analysis, and measuring the effect of changes in care. The CNL is expected to impact the quality of care at the microsystem level by measuring and monitoring outcomes. In order to accomplish this expectation the curriculum must include course work and learning opportunities in setting outcomes and outcomes assessment. Skill in data analysis and drawing conclusions from data is important.

Advocacy is an important role for the CNL. The CNL advocates for patients and their families and members of the healthcare team. Because of the CNL's system focus, he or she may have the fullest and most accurate understanding of issues that need to be addressed and mechanisms to address them. Content and learning experiences for building advocacy skills are usually integrated or woven through CNL courses. However, important content to include is communication theory, negotiation theory, conflict management, and ethics in health care.

One way to serve as a patient advocate is providing patient education services and measuring the outcomes. Clients today require in-depth, up-to-date knowledge about themselves, their health status, and treatment options. The CNL curriculum contains comprehensive content on educating clients and families—not just on how to perform a procedure at home but also the nature of the problem, and how they can acquire additional knowledge about the condition and support from others with similar problems. Health literacy assessment is critical to any teaching plan. Clients today must become independent managers of their own care. In some situations, referrals to advanced practice nurses or other healthcare professionals is most appropriate. Critical content would include understanding the scope and role for advanced practice nurses, teaching learning principles, consultation, program development, and evaluation.

Another crucial aspect of advocacy is working with intra- and interdisciplinary teams. In order for care to be client-centered, the client's needs and wishes must be at the forefront of decision making by any member of the health team. Integrating client-centered care requires that the healthcare team discuss the client's problem and agree on a common course of action. The CNL has the most comprehensive knowledge about the client's needs as well as current evidence related to the client's needs. Given this context, the CNL is the most logical provider for coordinating the team. The CNL has the opportunity to engage all members of the healthcare team during the academic program to improve continuity of care, safety, effectiveness, and coordination, leading to overall better outcomes and lower costs associated with care. The CNL role was specifically designed to have a major impact on reducing risks and increasing efficiency through systems analysis. Systematic analytical thinking is a critical skill for the CNL to ensure client safety and improve healthcare outcomes. These skills provide the opportunity for the CNL to link processes with patterns, thus making important connections. Content and learning experiences include systems theory, complexity theory, and communication theory. The ability to synthesize effective communication, decision-making, and critical thinking skills by CNL graduates is fundamental to their role of managing care of diverse and vulnerable patient groups.

To be effective in the CNL role, the graduate must be able to access, manage, evaluate, and use information systems and technology. The CNL must also be able

Figure 13-3 Safety and quality outcomes management assignment.

As a CNL, you will need access to in-depth information related to safety and quality outcomes management. An abundance of information can be found on the Internet, from pertinent articles to organizations concerned about safety and quality, to government entities that will assess an organization's commitment to delivering quality health care.

For this assignment, create a Webliography of 8–10 Web sites related to safety and quality outcomes management. Go to the top of the course Web page and locate the Webliography icon. Click on the icon, upload your Web sites, and provide a brief explanation of each site that includes why you believe the site will benefit you in your CNL practice. Be sure to save the Web sites on your own computer for personal future reference. Please do not use the links that were provided in the lecturette, but locate your own. Multiple sites exist.

Grading Rubric

____/5 points: 8–10 Web sites that relate to safety and quality improvement; useful to the CNL role.

____/6: Web site selection is original and creative, evidencing a thorough review of options.

____/9: Site descriptions are current, appropriately paraphrased, and cited in text and in reference list.

____/5: Correct use of APA style, grammar, spelling, punctuation, and word choice.

to assist other healthcare team members to incorporate new and evolving technologies as decision supports to improving client care outcomes. The curriculum must develop students' skills in using information systems and technologies so that knowledge is readily accessible at the point of care. Data not only guide plans of care but are also classified and stored for retrieval, analysis, and integration into evidence-based practice across the nation and across the world. The CNL graduate must be highly skilled in data management to facilitate essential changes in health care. Information becomes knowledge, and knowledge guides wise, thoughful decisions.

The influence of CNLs on the microsystems of interdisciplinary health care incorporates the perspectives of social justice, fiscal stewardship, client advocacy, and evidence-based practice. In the curriculum, the CNL will acquire the knowledge and skills to assume accountability for a designated population's quality healthcare outcomes and assume a horizontal leadership role in the healthcare team. CNL students must be able to analyze outcome-based measures and clinical guidelines to organize professional nursing care for health promotion and maintenance, prevention of illness, and rehabilitation of patients within the healthcare system. The ability to appraise strategies for collaboration with interdisciplinary health team members and culturally diverse consumers to advocate for patients and promote quality health care will improve the overall quality of care and the environment in which care is provided.

As previously stated, the CNL is not an administrator, and in many organizations the CNL will report to the unit manager. The CNL is, however, a team manager. Described as the "go-to" person on the clinical unit for clinical issues, within nursing or on an interdisciplinary basis, the CNL must be able to develop a highly functional team. This essential skill requires knowledge of group theory, delegation, horizontal leadership, fiscal management, team building, conflict management, and motivational theory.

Faculty must provide CNL students opportunities to analyze and evaluate actual CNL practice patterns. Courses that focus on building the students' competence in clinical decision making, problem identification, resource management, and outcome measurement for a selected patient population at the point of care are critical to full development of the competencies.

The clinical preparation of the CNL must include opportunities that provide in-depth experiences in the care of diverse populations, which are central to the educational program. These courses will foster the CNL's ability to assimilate and apply evidence-based information in the design, implementation, and evaluation of plans of care for individuals and cohorts. The CNL must be socialized to assume a leadership role in providing, managing, and evaluating patient care. The CNL collaborates with interdisciplinary health team members and consumers to advocate for patients and promote quality health care. This leadership and collaboration form the basis for CNL participation in policy formulation designed to meet patients' current and emerging needs. Further, the CNL can become an effective change agent and inspire changes in health care based on evidence.

In the clinician role, the CNL is expected to provide care to individuals and families at the point of care. Because the CNL is an advanced generalist, he or she will be expected to be able to deliver high quality care to a variety of patients and patient groups. The curriculum must offer the student the ability to develop the requisite knowledge and skills to allow the CNL to function at a high clinical level while simultaneously projecting leadership to elevate the care provided by all nurses in the facility. Necessary courses will include Advanced Pathophysiology, Advanced Pharmacology, and Physical Assessment Across the Life Span. Additionally, courses such as Evidence-Based Practice, Health Policy, and Finance are included to offer a strong basis for future skills development.

In our current cost-conscious environment, requesting more resources to support a failing system, especially when no one has reviewed the system to eliminate redundancies, is not likely to be supported. The CNL can lead the charge toward accountability and good fiscal stewardship of all healthcare resources as a condition of providing high-quality care. The CNL must understand the fiscal context of the practice site and be able to identify high-cost/high-volume activities in order to structure good return on investment. Basic business skills and organization theory can guide the developing CNL student in understanding economies of scale, reading balance sheets, differentiating between fixed and incremental costs, and implementing cost-effective measures to improve care.

The quality of practice is, to a large extent, measured by outcomes of client care. The CNL will be evaluated on his or her ability to improve care and cost outcomes in individuals and groups within clinical settings. Outcomes such as reducing recidivism in congestive heart failure patients, reducing hospital length of stay for clients with pneumonia or other infections, and improving participation in community outreach programs targeting keeping people well are examples of critical patient and systems outcomes.

The CNL must be provided with opportunities to differentiate between the clinical and cost outcomes that improve safety, effectiveness, timeliness, efficiency, quality, and patient-centered care. A part of that responsibility is emphasizing common clinical conditions that comprise a large part of healthcare activity and costs to determine where professional nursing practice can have the largest impact on outcomes. An example would be wellness programs targeting seniors with chronic conditions to help keep them healthy and reduce the financial costs associated with their care.

Students in the CNL program need to be involved in community-based, patient-centered projects, working with community health advisors, focused on the following core concepts:

1. *Dignity and Respect*: listening to and honoring patient and family perspectives and choices. Patient and family knowledge, values, beliefs, and cultural backgrounds are incorporated into the planning and delivery of care.

Figure 13-4 Threaded discussion on communication and relationship building.

This threaded discussion will assist you in considering the essential nature of communication and relationship building to the CNL roles, evidencing the often crucial and sometimes difficult conversations that are necessary to leadership and change. Senge (1990) describes shaping a culture of reflectiveness and deeper conversation—that is, creating change through conversation (p. 259).

Patterson, Grenny, McMillian, Switzler, and Sarton (2002) define a crucial conversation as a discussion (perhaps dialogue) between two or more people in which (1) stakes are high, (2) opinions vary, and (3) emotions run high (p. 3). Such crucial conversations might involve critiquing a colleague's work, giving feedback about behavior, giving an unfavorable performance review, or "pushing through" a major system's change. Participative openness and reflective openness can be considered aspects of these crucial conversations and transformative relationships. "Reflective openness leads to looking inward, allowing our conversations to make us more aware of the biases and limitations in our own thinking, and how our thinking and actions contribute to problems" (p. 261). Understanding this concept deepens our appreciation of mental models. Reflective openness, mental models, connectedness, and interdependency lead to transformative relationships. Understanding difficult conversations and one's "part" can give one greater influence in the change process.

Use this threaded discussion to dissect a crucial conversation that occurred during your immersion experience. What are you "hearing" in the conversation? What are you "seeing" in the conversation? What is not heard or seen that one might expect? What are the expectations? Were they met? If not, why not? If so, how did you know? Were outcomes met?

Please use the following grading rubric for completing your thread assignment:

____/5: Response is comprehensive, organized, and evidences a logical progression of ideas; effort and attention to detail is evident; communicates effectively all aspects of the discussion.

____/3: Supportive arguments, evidence, examples, and details are literature based and appropriately cited.

____/3: Response is original and creative, evidencing a thorough review of the literature related to the topic. Duplication of peer work, which already appears in threaded response, is minimal.

____/1: Sources cited in text and in reference list are current, appropriately paraphrased, and acknowledged.

____/1: Correct usage of APA style, grammar, spelling, punctuation, and word choice is evident.

2. *Information Sharing*: communicating complete and unbiased information with patients and families. This will facilitate continuity and comprehensiveness of care. Patients and families must receive timely, complete, and accurate information in order to effectively participate in care and decision making. The CNL student applies decision-making models and uses decision aids to empower patient and family decision making on health care and healthy lifestyle choices. Building and sustaining therapeutic relationships with patients and families is essential to the provision of high-quality, patient-centered care.

3. *Collaboration*: involving community partners, patients, and families on a community-wide basis. CNLs collaborate with healthcare leaders, patients, and families in policy and program development, implementation, and evaluation in healthcare facility design; and in professional education as well as care delivery. The CNL's leadership is key to protecting and promoting the health of citizens and communities. The CNL will assume responsibility for differences in clinical outcomes among diverse groups and can implement strategies that truly resolve disparities and the unequal distribution of healthcare resources.

In an online program preparing CNLs, threaded discussions can provide an opportunity to "see the situation" through the student's eyes. This can offer faculty a method of assessing interactions.

Patient-centered care is underscored in the CNL role. The Institute for Family-Centered Care identifies principles that guide the achievement of patient-centered care in hospitals of the future, as well as community-based care, including the following: addressing barriers to patient and family engagement such as low health literacy and personal and cultural preferences; eliminating disparities in the quality of care for minorities, the poor, the aged, and the mentally ill; improving the quality of care for the chronically ill through adoption of care models that encourage coordinated, multidisciplinary care; and using robust process improvement tools to improve quality and safety, and support achievement of patient-centered care. CNLs can make unique contributions to these settings by planning and implementing intervention strategies designed to facilitate care, eliminate barriers to care, and address the major lifestyle and environmental factors that contribute to premature morbidity and mortality.

Toward the end of their program of study, CNL students need opportunities to perform workflow analyses. An example of a workflow assignment is provided.

Figure 13-5 Workflow assignment.

The CNL uses the clinical immersion experience to assess, design, and implement a project plan. The experience culminates in evaluating outcomes from this work. Time spent in various activities, such as workflow assessment, gap analysis, interviewing, exploration of best practices, outlining measurement indicators, implementing intervention(s), evaluating and analyzing outcomes, provide the core work for the clinical work. Detailing this work, the following is to be considered. The workflow analysis provides the data required to develop the project plan and will be a summary report, providing documentation for the project plan.

_____/20 points: Workflow assessment (consider tools within the organization, accreditation bodies)

_____/15: Gap analysis (consider best practices, evidence-based guidelines)
  a. Use practice guidelines, best practices, and accreditation standards to compare current practices within unit, system, and so forth.
  b. Quantify data from workflow assessment and gap analysis (wait times, incident reports, medication error, infection rate, fall rate, complications, etc.)

_____/20: Interview individuals from work involved in workflow and gap analysis (use a variety of guides from the literature)
  a. Major stakeholders (PI, CM, risk management, The Joint Commission representative, chief financial officer, etc.)
  b. Key individuals, including nurses and physicians
  c. Patients and families
  d. Qualitative data analysis

_____/15: Document your observational experiences (observing work flow on the unit/department)
  a. Patient admissions
  b. Patient care delivery
  c. Patient discharges
  d. Patient transfers

Describe your experiences in a drop-box assignment. Prior to submitting the assignment for a grade, please confer with your CNL preceptor. Share the outcomes of the conference in your assignment. Also, please describe the impact of this experience on your learning.

In addition to being direct care providers, the CNL is accountable for the care outcomes of clinical populations or a specified group of clients in a healthcare system. As clinical decision maker and care manager, the CNL coordinates the direct care activities of other nursing staff and health professionals. The CNL provides lateral integration of care services within a microsystem of care to effect quality, client-care outcomes. To prepare students for the CNL role, there must be a deliberate and integrated inclusion of leadership education and socialization that begins on the first day of the first class and continues throughout the CNL education program. For example, leadership content should be incorporated in every client care plan prepared by students so that each plan includes not only clinical actions for meeting the needs of the client but also an organizational plan for delegation of care to assisting personnel, registered nurses, and other health professionals, including the teaching and evaluation activities that would need to accompany such delegation. One leadership course taken in the last year of the CNL course of study is not sufficient to prepare the student who can perform as a beginning CNL upon graduation. Practice at the unit and systems level will require a shift in thinking on the faculty's part, with greater attention to context and the development of leadership skills throughout the curriculum. Students, as well, may have to be convinced that systems-level intervention, such as the implementation of best practices and the revision of guidelines and protocols for the management of clinical populations, is essential for professional practice and has a greater probability of generating superior and far-reaching outcomes.

The immersion experience focuses on team leading and building, advocacy, communication, resource and outcomes management, and evidence-based practice. Implement evidence-based nursing care to ensure that patients benefit from the latest knowledge and innovation in health care. CNL students learn to apply leadership, care management, and teaching skills to oversee the care coordination of a distinct group of patients and provide direct patient care in complex situations. Specifically, the CNL is educated in clinical leadership and is able to implement outcome-based practice and quality improvement strategies. The CNL role is responsible for creation and management of microsystems of care that are responsive to the healthcare needs of individuals and families.

As discussions occur among the CNL, faculty, preceptors, and others on the units, new opportunities for improvement emerge and are shared, and change is tested, with more new opportunities surfacing through the process. The following are examples of course titles from schools offering CNL preparation: Clinical Nurse

Figure 13-6 CNL course titles and examples.

MSN 6400 Quality Management of the Environment (3 credits)

Based on organizational theory, students are introduced to the healthcare system as a laterally integrated care environment. The current *National Patient Safety Goals*, the Institute of Medicine (IOM) indicators of quality patient care, and evidence-based practice are essential components of an environmental culture that promotes quality and provides the framework for the course. The course highlights the communication, collaboration, consultation, and leadership skills needed to enhance the student's ability to question and analyze clinical issues and enhance clinical judgments. The relationship of safe quality care to effective delegation and clinical resource utilization will be analyzed. The course emphasizes the role of the clinical nurse leader as a leader, educator, and advocate for safe, cost-effective, quality care.

MSN 6401 Practicum 1: Quality Management of the Environment (Practicum) (1 credit)

This course provides for initiation into the CNL role in a care setting in which management of clinical systems and national patient safety goals can be assessed and evaluated. Students learn to serve as both leader and partner on an interdisciplinary healthcare team in a selected clinical site. Emphasis is placed on the integration of theory and research discussed in earlier courses and the organization and leadership theory presented in MSN 6400. The student will select and describe a focused clinical problem that would have implications for improvement in clinical patient outcomes. Students begin to learn to effectively delegate and manage nursing resources.

Source: From Curry College Faculty. Master's CNL curriculum. Elizabeth C. Kudzma, DNSc, MPH, Professor, MSN Program Director, Division of Nursing, Curry College; Linda M. Caldwell, DNSc, Professor, Nursing Chairperson, Curry College; Linda Tenofsky, PhD, Professor, Basic Program Coordinator.

Leader Quality and Safety, Clinical Decision Making and Advanced Health Assessment, Health Promotion and Disease Prevention, Evidence-Based Practice, Healthcare Quality, Principles of Clinical Outcomes Management, Organizational Dynamics, Program Planning, Business of Health Care, Economics and Policy in Health Care, Philosophical and Ethical Issues, Leadership, and CNL Advocacy and Education.

CNL Education Tools

Content mapping is a useful tool that educators can use to ensure that all content is sufficiently covered when developing the new CNL curriculum. A grid is developed, and on the *Y* axis, the essential CNL content, as identified by the *CNL Curriculum Framework for Client-Centered Healthcare* (AACN, 2006a), is listed. On the *X* axis, the existing course or courses to be developed are listed and a cross-check is conducted to determine whether the content is present or to place content into courses under development.

Summary

- The CNL is educated in a master's in nursing program and is prepared as an advanced generalist.
- Quality, safety, and evidence-based practice are the cornerstones of CNL practice.
- Educational preparation for the CNL occurs at the master's level and builds on a liberal education foundation and the competencies for the baccalaureate in nursing.
- Faculty use the following references for developing a CNL program: *The Essentials for Master's Education for Advanced Practice Nursing* (AACN, 1996), *CNL Tool Kit* (AACN, 2006b), and AACN's *White Paper on the Education and Role of the Clinical Nurse Leader* (2007).
- All programs must prepare students to sit for certification, and therefore students are expected to have at least 500 clinical hours including a clinical immersion experience in the CNL.

Reflection Questions

1. What are the similarities in curricular models used to educate CNLs? What modifications could be made to improve outcomes?
2. Because faculty must be actively involved with clinical partners in assisting with the creation and implementation of the CNL role in their facilities, will this result in greater congruence between practice and education?

Learning Activity

1. Using the *CNL Framework for Client-Centered Healthcare* (AACN, 2006), analyze the CNL curriculum at your school to determine whether all elements are present.

Recommended Reading

Aiken, L. H., Clarke, S, P., Cheung, R. B., Sloane, D. M., & Silber, J. H. (2003). Educational levels of hospital nurses and surgical patient mortality. *Journal of the American Medical Association, 290*(12), 1617–1623.

American Association of Colleges of Nursing (AACN). (2008). *Clinical nurse leader (CNL) talking points*. Retrieved July 22, 2008, from http://www.aacn.nche.edu/cnl/docs/CNLTalking Points.doc

American Organization of Nurse Executives. (2004). *AONE guiding principles*. Retrieved February 12, 2008, from http://www.aone.org/aone/resource/guidingprinciples.html

Aspden, P., Corrigan, J. M., Wolcott, J., & Erickson, S. M. (Eds.). (2004). *Patient safety: Achieving a new standard for care*. Washington, DC. National Academy of Sciences.

Fitzpatrick, J. J., & Wallace, M. (2004). *The doctor of nursing practice and clinical nurse leader: Essentials of program development and implementation for clinical practice*. New York: Springer.

Harris, J. L., Tornabeni, J., & Walters, S. E. (2006). The clinical nurse leader: A valued member of the healthcare team. *Journal of Nursing Administration, 36*(10), 446–449.

Institute of Medicine (IOM). (1999). *To err is human: Building a safer health system*. Washington, DC: Institute of Medicine and National Academies Press.

Institute of Medicine (IOM). (2001a). *Crossing the quality chasm*. Washington, DC: National Academies Press. Retrieved February 22, 2008, from http://www.iom.edu/Object.File/Master/27/184/Chasm-8pager.pdf

Institute of Medicine (IOM). (2001b). *Envisioning the national health care quality*. Washington, DC: National Academies Press.

Institute of Medicine (IOM). (2002a). *Unequal treatment confronting racial and ethnic disparities in health*. Washington, DC: National Academies Press.

Institute of Medicine (IOM). (2002b). *Guidance for the national healthcare disparities report*. Washington, DC: National Academies Press.

Institute of Medicine (IOM). (2003a). *Priority areas for national action: Transforming health care quality*. Washington, DC: National Academies Press.

Institute of Medicine (IOM). (2003b). *Leadership by example: Coordinating government roles in improving health care*. Washington, DC: National Academies Press.

The Joint Commission. (2009). *2009 national patient safety goals*. Retrieved February 22, 2008, from http://www.jointcommission.org/patientsafety/nationalpatientsafetygoals

Lewis, J. (2006). *Fundamentals of project management.* (3rd ed.). New York: AMACOM.

Melnyk, B. M., & Fineout-Overholt, E. (Eds.). (2004). *Evidence-based practice in nursing & healthcare: A guide to best practice.* Philadelphia. Lippincott Williams & Wilkins.

Nelson, E., Baltadan, P., & Godfrey, M. (2007). *Quality by design: A clinical microsystem approach.* San Francisco: Jossey Bass.

Porter-O'Grady, T., & Malloch, K. (2007). *Managing for success in health care.* St Louis, MO: Elsevier.

Scalise, D. (2005). Patient care: The safety network. *Hospitals & Health Networks, 79*(12), 16–17.

References

American Association of Colleges of Nursing (AACN). (1996). *The essentials of master's education for advanced practice nursing.* Retrieved February 12, 2009, http://www.aacn.nche.edu/Education/pdf/MasEssentials96.pdf

American Association of College of Nursing (AACN). (2004). *Working statement comparing CNL and CNS roles: Similarities, differences & complementarities.* Retrieved April 27, 2009, from http://www.aacn.nche.edu/CNL/pdf/WorkingStatement.pdf

American Association of Colleges of Nursing (AACN). (2006a). *Preparing graduates for practice as a clinical nurse leader: Draft curriculum framework.* Retrieved June 23, 2009, from http://www.aacn.nche.edu/CNL/pdf/curricufrmwrk.pdf

American Association of Colleges of Nursing (AACN). (2006b). *Took kit for the implementation of the clinical nurse leader: Guide for practice and academic partners.* Retrieved June 23, 2009, from http://www.aacn.nche.edu/cnl/toolkit.htm

American Association of Colleges of Nursing (AACN). (2007). *White paper on the education and role of the clinical nurse leader.* Retrieved February 12, 2009, from http://www.aacn.nche.edu/Publications/WhitePapers/ClinicalNurseLeader07.pdf

Berwick, D., Godfrey, A., & Roessner, J. (2002). *Curing healthcare: New strategies for healthcare improvement.* Hoboken, NJ: Jossey-Bass/Wiley.

Bower, K. A. (2006). *Designing a care delivery model ... the what, the how, the CNL.* Presentation given at AACN Regional Conferences on Clinical Nurse Leader, Denver, CO.

Patterson, K., Grenny, J., McMillan, R., Switzler, A., & Sarton, M. (2002). *Crucial conversations: Tools for talking when stakes are high.* New York: McGraw-Hill.

Senge, P. (1990). *The fifth discipline: The art and practice of the learning organization.* New York: Doubleday.

FOURTEEN

Creative and Meaningful Clinical Immersions

■ Patricia L. Thomas and James L. Harris

■ **Learning Objectives**

- ■ Discuss why a needs assessment and gap analysis are important prior to the clinical immersion experience.
- ■ Discuss the importance of using business principles during the clinical immersion experience.
- ■ Discuss techniques and components to include when developing a portfolio of clinical experiences.
- ■ Discuss the impact of metrics when addressing needs and gaps during the immersion experience.

"There is only one thing stronger than all the armies in the world, and that is an idea whose time has come."

Victor Hugo

"Plans are nothing; planning is everything."

Dwight D. Eisenhower

Key Terms

Needs assessment	Gap analysis
Portfolio	Business principles
Planning	Metrics

CNL Roles

Clinician	Outcomes manager
Coordinator of care	Information manager
Lifelong learner	Team manager
Systems analyst/risk anticipator	

CNL Professional Values

Accountability	Fiscal stewardship
Outcome measurement	Microsystem management
Quality improvement	Evidence-based practice
Interdisciplinary teams	Quality patient care and safety

CNL Core Competencies

Communication	Assessment
Environment of care manager	Member of a profession
Team leader	Designer/manager/coordinator of care
Information and healthcare technologies	

Introduction

Meaningful and innovative clinical immersions for the clinical nurse leader (CNL) student are the culmination of academic and clinical experiences throughout a CNL program that can be limited when faculty, clinical partners, and students do not mutually identify needs and create developmental opportunities within a microsystem. Mutually identified clinical immersions for the CNL student should be based and focused on identifying and assessing gaps and needs within an organization while improving the health of a population of patients within a given microsystem. This critical point cannot be overstated. Without thoughtful planning that is detailed and deliberate, the clinical immersion experience can be a point of tension and opportunities for successful launching into the CNL role can be missed.

Nelson, Batalden, and Godfrey (2007) identified the importance of discovering the microsystem by studying its five Ps—purpose, patients, professionals, processes, and patterns—and the ways each of the parts interacts with another. The smallest measurable detail should be analyzed and iterative work redesign and learning cycles developed that result in changing work processes and developing database and feedback systems to the microsystem level. Thus, gaps between the unit and organizational levels are closed, improvement in the utility of information occurs, and a management focus that corresponds with the real work is created. The unit of work is therefore aligned with the unit of analysis and unit of intervention (Nelson et al., 2007; Linda Norman lecture, Vanderbilt University, 2007).

A meaningful clinical immersion is established when CNL students are able to integrate their course work into valued clinical work through the enactment of the CNL role. The clinical immersion experience is intended to provide the platform to support transformative learning, initially for the CNL student and the microsystem, and eventually for the organization. Transformative learning is described as the culmination of past experiences and perspectives joined with new learning to support resocialization that involves critical reflection of the learner's past and present perspectives to understand one's self and one's paradigm. Beliefs and old ways of thinking are examined and critical reflection is triggered, leading to alternative ways of thinking and acting. Within a clinical immersion experience, students are encouraged and supported in changing their worldview and role, internalizing new ways of thinking, communicating, and behaving, supported by a precepted clinical immersion experience in a microsystem (Mezirow, 1997; Morris & Faulk, 2007). Fundamental to early outcomes, clinical partners and students need to question assumptions, beliefs, and values, and consider multiple points of view while seeking to verify rationale for the clinical immersion experience (Bouchard, St-Jacques, Robillard, & Renaud, 2008; Stanley, Hoiting, Burton, Harris, & Norman, 2007; Mezirow, 1997).

Figure 14-1 Unit clinical project data and source worksheet.

Type of Data	Source of Data	Target and Compliance Percentage
Troponin level returned to provider for review and action within 60 minutes of order	Acute coronary syndrome performance measure *Balanced scorecard*	100/90
Percentage of patients who received smoking cessation at least once during inpatient admission	Smoking cessation performance measure; inpatient *Inpatient education tracking monitor*	80/50
Percentage of inpatients diagnosed with heart failure who received all five components of discharge instructions	Heart failure discharge instructions; inpatient *Balanced scorecard*	100/15

Using Data and Resources to Identify Needs and Craft Meaningful Clinical Immersion Experiences

A variety of data and resources are available for analysis at the microsystem level that corresponds to the CNL student's learning objectives. Examples include balanced scorecards, quality markers, performance and target measures, and patient and staff satisfaction scores. The identified microsystem gaps can be transformed into meaningful clinical immersion experiences and projects that develop CNL students, create additional examples of outcomes for their portfolio, and benefit the overall function of the unit. In examining unit data, CNL students can identify an area of interest to allow an innovative approach to issues that are easy recognized in the microsystem.

Upon identifying gaps, the CNL student can organize a clinical immersion project that meets the needs of the objectives in the clinical immersion course while addressing important concerns in the organization. Linking a microsystem issue or concern to the planning of the immersion project then benefits the student and orga-

---

Figure 14-2 Clinical project status summary.

Summary of Project:

Problems Encountered: Actions Taken:

1.   1.

2.   2.

Planned Activities for Next Reporting Period:

---

nization alike. Utilizing unit assessment tools provided in a didactic course offers the CNL a framework for analyzing opportunities in the microsystem. The assessment tool provides a springboard for specific problem identification that leads to quality improvement methodologies, team engagement, and team leader opportunities, and specific measure and metrics to demonstrate outcomes. This also creates additional examples of outcomes for the CNL's portfolio, and ultimately benefits patient care delivery and patient outcomes.

When establishing a project status summary, attention needs to be placed on the process and patterns students observe in terms of collaboration with the interdisciplinary team members, inclusion of staff in quality improvement initiatives, relationships established with departments or project champions in the organization, and the responses of patients, family, and staff. Because CNLs are expected to serve as the team or project leader, insights are gained as students reflect on their interactions and leadership skills are expanded.

The Business Model Applied to CNL Clinical Immersions

Uncontrollable issues in clinical settings may deter the development of innovative approaches to problem resolution and work redesign. Staff finds themselves performing multiple tasks, getting trapped in existent business models and processes that are ineffective and obsolete. Without insight, the CNL student clinical immersion experiences may be less than meaningful and lack innovation that demonstrates the incorporation and integration of advances of new technologies and methods (Hwang & Christensen, 2008). So how can the elements of a business model guide a CNL clinical immersion experience?

According to Hwang and Christensen (2008), all business models consist of three components: a value proposition, resources and processes, and a profit formula. The value proposition is the service (quality and safe patient care) that assists individuals to accomplish desired goals and objectives. In order to be successful, resources must be dedicated that include expert and knowledgeable staff, engagement of academic partners, and equipment necessary to provide care. Processes are identified that ensure activities and actions are developed and initiated that result in desired outcomes and are framed for data capture and future trending. The final component is the profit formula, in which any organization determines the price and benefits that can be sustained over time. Organizations can use this model as other services are envisioned and ultimately offered. The CNL student and the assigned preceptor can use this as a road map in developing the clinical immersion experience.

The CNL student can facilitate the development of the project and plan with clinicians and managers to develop a cost-benefit analysis in concert with course objectives. This project can continue throughout the entire clinical immersion. An example of a clinical immersion experience for a CNL student that incorporates each of the three components of the business model is illustrated in Figure 14-3.

The Utility of Portfolios

A professional portfolio is a summary and history of collected documents that showcases accomplishments. It also demonstrates how various elements of a professional's role functions are related, highlighting competence and development of a role over time (Billings & Kowalski, 2008; Sherrod, 2005). From the beginning courses in a CNL program, students should collect documents from assigned classroom activities and save examples of their writing and accomplishments. The examples become the tool kit that can be shared with prospective employers to demonstrate accomplishments on a résumé and to show that academic knowledge has been translated into meaningful actions and interventions that can be used to improve a microsystem. Upon graduation, the portfolio is used to persuade an employer or supervisor that the CNL can enact the CNL *End-of-Program Competencies* (defined by the AACN,

Figure 14-3 Clinical immersion project: Medical/psychiatric unit.

Value Proposition	Resources and Processes	Profit Formula
Medical/psychiatric unit dedicated to comprehensive care for patients requiring acute and chronic medical and psychiatric interventions by an interdisciplinary team skilled in medical and psychiatric care	Unit design and construction, staff development, equipment purchase and staff training, and marketing strategies that includes patient education materials	Cost/benefit analysis that includes all start-up costs and savings by a comprehensive unit that eliminates transfer of psychiatric patients with acute and chronic medical problems of a medical unit that historically required 1:1 sitters

2006) and that the student has experience to support what is claimed on his or her résumé.

The portfolio presented at the fruition of a clinical immersion experience chronicles the process and evidence utilized to successfully complete the capstone project. Inherent to the portfolio document for the clinical immersion are a detailed plan that identifies the microsystem problem to be addressed, project objectives, deliverables, timelines, and data or metrics. Less evident to an untrained eye are the redesign efforts undertaken to improve clinical outcomes of care for the population of the microsystem and the leadership efforts required to guide an interdisciplinary team to success.

Aside from the information related to your education, licensure, work experience, and certifications, the following are additional tips for creating effective portfolio designs (Elbow and Belanoff, 1997):

- Create a well-designed cover.
- Place information behind tabs to organize the content.
- Use colorful charts or graphics to demonstrate impact or outcomes achieved.
- Include examples that illustrate cost savings and innovations.

Performance Contracts

As CNLs graduate and accept positions, the performance contract is a common mechanism to define the role expectations and markers of impact and success. The portfolio

Figure 14-4 Clinical nurse leader performance contract.

Rating Period: _____–_____		
Name: _____	**Unit Assigned:** _____	
Measure	**Target**	**Comments From Quarterly Review**
Infectious Disease: Blood cultures collected before administration of first antibiotic.	93%	
Immunizations: Patients received immunization during flu season (_____–_____)	90%	
Inpatient Satisfaction: Evidence of satisfied inpatients during each stay.	85%	

_____/_____   _____

Clinical nurse leader/Supervisor   Date

documentation serves as a quick reference to prospective employers about past performance and what can be expected in the future. An example of a performance contract is shown in Figure 14-4.

Measurement for CNL Success

The challenge for the CNL student and those in practice is to design methods that measure impact and clinical outcomes that are sustainable. Nelson et al. (2007) stated that measurement is forward progress and clinical leaders functioning within the microsystem must engage all teams of staff to be innovative, creative, and participatory in the improvement of healthcare delivery. Didactic course work and clinical immersions must prepare CNL students to understand and collaboratively develop measurement tools that are applicable to the practice environment. Within all microsystems are numerous data points waiting to be mined, analyzed, and displayed. Creating an area to display data as a "data board" allows the CNL to visually demonstrate each metric for the members of the microsystem to observe. This is a key role for the CNL. The data should represent the current value or target and the impacts over a period of time. This information can drive clinical and quality improvements and identify other improvement projects necessary to meet organizational goals, regulatory requirements, and specific microsystem improvement that ultimately enhance quality and delivery of care.

But how does the CNL identify appropriate metrics? A starting point is to review unit goals, the population served, and the services provided. The microsystem model with its five Ps—professionals, patients, philosophy, processes, patterns—may also provide assessment data for the identification outcomes and measures. For example, a CNL assigned to a long-term care area may focus on increasing residents' functional status by measuring involvement in daily activities offered by staff. The CNL assigned to ambulatory surgery units can measure the number of cancellations and the financial impacts incurred by each cancellation. This can be further measured and trended by service or product. The information can then be used by project improvement teams to develop strategies and tactics to improve efficiency. These are only two of the many projects CNLs can measure and have an impact on to enhance both financial and quality outcomes within a microsystem.

Summary

- CNL clinical experiences must be creatively developed, meaningful to the student, and value-added for the organization.
- Multiple data and other resources are readily available for CNL students to access when developing a clinical immersion project.
- The business case for a CNL project must be supported by outcomes and evidence-based data.
- Portfolios of CNL projects can be valuable to the healthcare facility when displaying quality outcomes, partnerships with academic affiliates, and for the CNL when applying for positions.
- A performance contract is a method useful to the CNL and the organization when tracking successes and identifying opportunities for improvement.

Reflection Questions

1. What part of the clinical immersion project do you feel most prepared for? Least prepared for?
2. What are the critical elements of a clinical immersion project?
3. What resources do you have assist you in completing the clinical immersion?
4. What documents do you have that demonstrate your skills and accomplishments for the CNL role?

Learning Activities

1. Gather documents to create a professional portfolio. Consider how you will organize the information. Share your ideas and documents with a classmate to perform peer review.
2. Have students divide into groups of two or three. Ask them to brainstorm about assignments that have been completed that would be appropriate for inclusion in their portfolio.
3. Bring a project plan for a completed project to class. The project plan should include a timeline with detailed action steps, contact persons/responsible parties, and deliverables. Describe how a project plan for your clinical immersion would be different from previous project plans.

Recommended Reading

American Association of Colleges of Nursing (AACN). (2007, July). *White paper on the education and role of the Clinical Nurse Leader*. Available at http://www.aacn.nche.edu/ Publications/WhitePapers/ClinicalNurseLeader07.pdf

Elbow, P., & Belanoff, P. (1997). Reflections on an explosion: Portfolios in the 90's and beyond. In K. Yancey & J. Weiser (Eds.), *Situating portfolios: Four perspectives* (pp. 21–23). Logan, UT: Utah State University Press.

References

American Association of Colleges of Nursing (AACN). (2006, May). *End-of-program competencies & required clinical experiences for the Clinical Nurse Leader*. Available at http://www.aacn.nche.edu/CNL/pdf/EndCompsgrid.pdf

Billings, D., & Kowalski, K. (2008). Developing your career as a nurse educator: The professional portfolio. *Journal of Continuing Education in Nursing, 39*(12), 532–533.

Bourchard, S., St-Jacques, J., Robillard, G., & Renaud, P. (2008). Anxiety increases the feeling of presence in virtual reality. *Presence, 17*(4), 376–391.

Hwang, J., & Christensen, C. M. (2008). Technology: New technologies demand new business models. In Society for Healthcare Strategy and Market Development (Ed.), *FutureScan: Healthcare trends and implications 2008–2013.* Chicago: Health Administration Press.

Mezirow, J. (1997). Transformative learning: Theory to practice. *New Directions for Adult and Continuing Education. 74,* 5–12.

Morris, A. H. & Faulk, D. (2007). Perspective transformation: Enhancing the development of professionalism in the RN-to-BSN students. *Journal of Nursing Education, 46*(10), 445–451.

Nelson, E. C., Batalden, P. B., & Godfrey, M. M. (2007). *Quality by design: A clinical microsystems approach.* San Francisco: Jossey-Bass.

Sherrod, D. (2005). The professional portfolio: A snapshot of your career. *Nursing Management, 36*(9), 74–75.

Stanley, J M., Hoiting, T., Burton, T., Harris, J., & Norman, L. (2007). Implementing innovation through education-practice partnerships. *Nursing Outlook, 55*(2), 67–73.

——————— Unit 7 ———————

Initiating and Sustaining the Clinical Nurse Leader Role: A Practical Guide

FIFTEEN

Strategies for CNL Inclusion in a Model of Care Delivery for a Multihospital System

■ Joan Shinkus Clark

■ **Learning Objectives**

> ■ Identify insights into implementation of the CNL role in the context of model for care delivery congruent with the organization's foundation for nursing practice.

> "You must be the change you wish to see in the world."
>
> Mahatma Gandhi

> ■ Describe guidelines for implementation of a care delivery model that features the role of the CNL across the organization.

Key Terms

Career pathways
12-Bed Hospital
Business case

Models of care delivery
Team manager

CNL Roles

Outcome manager
Educator
Team manager
Lifelong learner

Client advocate
Systems analysis/risk anticipator
Member of a profession

CNL Professional Values

Altruism
Human dignity
Social justice

Accountability
Integrity

CNL Core Competencies

Critical thinking
Ethics
Global health care
Provider and manager of care
Nursing technology and resource
  management

Communication
Human diversity
Healthcare systems and policy
Designer/manager/coordinator of care
Member of a profession

Introduction

Experience teaches us that it takes a vision of the CNL role as the linchpin for a broader strategy or model for care delivery. It is in that broader context that the CNL role becomes embraced, and then embedded, into a broader strategy of creating strong clinical career pathways to retain and engage nursing staff in a culture of lifelong learning. In this chapter, a nurse executive chronicles an experience with implementing new care delivery models focused around the concept of the CNL. The experience began before the definition of the CNL role and has evolved into care delivery model development in multiple settings and sites. Described here is one approach to implementing the CNL role in the context of a larger model, based on landmark work with the 12-Bed Hospital in Miami, Florida, and the evolution to implementing a delivery model in a healthcare system with 14 hospitals ranging from 36 to 866 beds.

Background

The story begins in the early years of the 21st century, when the healthcare world was awakening from the aftermath of the reengineering craze of the 1990s. This was a time when hospital care became "patient focused," assisted by cross-trained support staff, ready to serve patients their meals, clean up their rooms, and also provide personal care, all by the same person! In addition, nurse managers expanded their accountability to multiple departments within their facilities, as well as functions. Suddenly managers were learning the intricacies of supervising room cleaning and the details that go along with housekeeping, to say nothing about other services, such as respiratory therapy, admitting, patient transport, meal delivery, and the like. Nurses were picking up any slack in this ambitious care model, and the strain was beginning to show.

As a new chief nursing officer (CNO) at Baptist Hospital of Miami, a 577-bed hospital, the author began at a time when dissatisfaction with this situation was at its height. Nursing turnover had increased as support for delivery of patient care had diminished and dissatisfaction with the delivery model increased. In the initial months in the facility, it was painfully apparent that the model was not sustainable and nurses were leaving because their concerns about the model were going unheard. To begin the dialogue toward a remedy for this situation, staff on each unit were asked to determine their ideal staffing pattern in a facilitated two-day process called "Fastrack." Parameters for their decision making were provided, including reaching a consensus on which of the support services they wanted to recentralize. A commitment was communicated to abide by their recommendations, as long as they were within the given parameters.

When the staff on the 52-bed cardiovascular unit made their recommendations, involved in the staffing mix was a role that would act as a clinical leader for a team of about a dozen patients. It was important to the staff that the leader not be responsible for management functions; rather, his or her primary purpose would be to act as a patient navigator and a central point for communication among other team members. The patient oversight would be limited to about 12 patients, so the nurse could realistically follow each patient and have enough time to adequately stay on top of critical issues. The individual would be a role model and expert, and although not taking an actual assignment, he or she would play a backup role for the other nurses in their 12-bed area.

Once the basic blueprint for the position was described and was supported by the director of nursing for that division, the author's support was requested. The author asked that a job description be developed for the role. The staff named the role *patient care facilitator* (PCF; see Appendix A for job description). Qualifications for the PCF included a baccalaureate degree in nursing, 3–5 years' clinical experience, expert role model, and a willingness to assume 24-hour accountability for the patients in their assigned geographical area. The hours of work were Monday through Friday on the day shift which allowed the role some flexibility around working the hours most appropriate for the type of specialty and unit.

The nursing director used a vacant position that was available to initiate the pilot, and within weeks of choosing a baccalaureate-prepared nurse on the unit and implementing the pilot project, it was apparent that the new role was making a big impact on the staff, the patients, and physicians. Over the next few months, indicators such as patient satisfaction, patient safety goal follow-through, and core measure improvements were providing additional validation that this role was making a difference. The nursing director for the cardiovascular unit began to recruit for additional PCFs to complete coverage for the remaining 12-bed sections, and over the next 6 months, reports about this new role spread across the nursing units.

When the nursing director for the medical-surgical units approached the author with a proposal to implement the PCF role on two additional units, the intention was to implement four PCF roles on each department at the same time. This initiative was to expedite improvements, particularly in patient satisfaction. There were sufficient vacancies in these departments that most of the additions to the indirect care hours could be absorbed, so the proposal was approved. In order to assure consistency with the selection and orientation of new PCFs to the other departments, a project manager was assigned. The project manager was one of the staff on the original unit that first described the PCF role and developed the job description. It was determined that new PCFs would be mentored by incumbent PCFs, first in the experienced PCF's department and then as part of the team on the new PCF's unit, to assure role consistency.

12-Bed Hospital

At the end of that year, the author was asked to provide the keynote speech for the annual retreat for nursing leadership, and it was suggested that the speech focus on the progress of the PCF pilot project on the three nursing units. In preparation for presentation, it was hard to describe the gestalt of the experience by simply describing the project in terms of the new role that had been described. Contemplating the role, there was consideration of traditional models of care delivery and it was noted that there were elements of many of these models in the context of the role being piloted. Figure 15-1 depicts the traditional care delivery models and how they relate to the PCF role.

It was noted that this was not just a new role, but in its definition at the 12- to 16-bed level, it was actually a care model. In the implementation of the role, all attempts were made to keep the same staff together within the PCF's assigned geography. In this way, the synergy of a high-performing team would be more likely to occur. The conclusion was that the model evolving around this role was a little bit of the most common nursing care models. The term *12-Bed Hospital* emerged as a model that made a difference by breaking the patient unit into small, manageable segments, under the care of a clinical leader.

With the presentation at the retreat, the concept of the 12-Bed Hospital cast around the role of the PCF resonated with the group in attendance, and other specialty area managers spoke to how the model could work in many of the specialty units as well. The hospital CEO was also in attendance and, witnessing the synergy around this model, he offered his support to a hospital-wide implementation over the next two budget years.

By 2004, all areas of the hospital had implemented the 12-Bed Hospital model, with the exception of the outpatient and short-stay units, the PACU, labor and delivery, inpatient rehabilitation, and the interventional suite. Some of the PCFs

Figure 15-1   12-Bed Hospital as a model of care delivery.

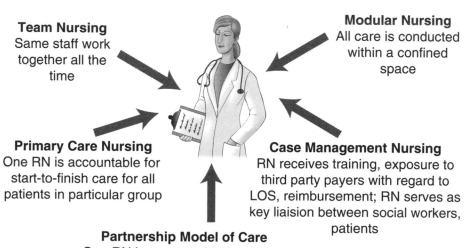

12-BED CARE MODEL INCORPORATES BEST ATTRIBUTES
OF TRADITIONAL NURSING PRACTICES/DELIVERY MODELS

Team Nursing
Same staff work
together all the
time

Modular Nursing
All care is conducted
within a confined
space

Primary Care Nursing
One RN is accountable for
start-to-finish care for all
patients in particular group

Case Management Nursing
RN receives training, exposure to
third party payers with regard to
LOS, reimbursement; RN serves as
key liaision between social workers,
patients

Partnership Model of Care
One RN is accountable for care of
patient for shift and partners with other
licenses and non-licensed caregivers

were interested in educational advancement, or were already master's prepared as an advanced practice nurse, so an advanced patient care facilitator job description was developed to allow for additional clinical advancement (Shinkus Clark, 2004).

Also in 2007, the American Association of Colleges of Nursing (AACN) published their original White Paper on the role of the clinical nurse leader. Coincidental to Baptist Hospital's first dissemination of results of the first few years' experience with their model, a role called the clinical nurse leader, very similar in function, was also being described, but prepared at the master's level of education. After presentation of the 12-Bed Hospital model nationally at the ANCC Magnet Conference, as well as the AONE Annual Meeting, Baptist began getting inquiries and requests for site visits, as other organizations began to evaluate changes to their models. Internally, the creators of this model began to follow the events occurring nationally related to the CNL, as opposed to our concept of the advanced PCF, which accommodated for the CNS and the ARNP. The creators of the model aligned the advanced practice model around the PCF role to provide 24-hour support for patients. The idea of encouraging PCFs to pursue CNL education began to resonate.

In 2005, Baptist Hospital and the Christine E. Lynn College of Nursing at the Florida Atlantic University (FAU) in Boca Raton, Florida, formalized a service-education partnership and BHM provided scholarships for 11 of their PCFs for their CNL program. The partnership model proved to be beneficial for the overall synergy in the classroom. PCFs spoke from an experiential point of view to form class discussion and at the same time, benefited from a curriculum specifically designed to enhance competencies they needed for the role (Sherman, Shinkus Clark, & Maloney, 2008). In March 2006, Baptist and FAU presented their partnership and highlighted the 12-Bed Hospital model for the national CNL forum via teleconference, providing the early adopters of the CNL role around the country with an overview of an organizational model for the nurse leader role.

In 2007, Health Workforce Solutions and the Robert Wood Johnson Foundation studied 24 promising models of care delivery, highlighting the 12-Bed Hospital as one of the top five models (Morjikian, Kimball, & Joynt, 2007). Of the 24 most promising models studied, the following key findings characterized the models:

- Elevated roles for nurses: nurses as care integrators
- Migration to interdisciplinary care: team approach
- Bridged continuum of care
- Pushed boundaries: for example, home as a setting of care
- Targeted high users of health care: elderly plus
- Sharpened focus on the patient
- Leveraged technology in care delivery
- Driven by results: improving satisfaction, quality, and cost

In the 12-Bed Hospital, all of these elements were to some degree integrated into the model. The PCF, APCF, and the CNL act as *care integrators* for the patient, family, and the rest of the healthcare team. As part of a clinical career pathway, nurses are able to advance educationally, yet have career opportunities that allow them to remain at the front line, doing patient care. Because they become the focal point for communication and planning for the patient, their care is team oriented, involving an *interdisciplinary approach.*

Although the roles were primarily assigned on the inpatient unit, patients and families along *the continuum* often maintained contact with the PCF after discharge.

Patients with chronic conditions that necessitated frequent hospital admissions often became "regulars" for an individual PCF. Many of the patients who benefited most by PCF, APCF, or CNL care were the *elderly*, especially those with multiple comorbidities and frequent emergency room visits and inpatient stays.

Among the intervening factors that prompted the emergence of the PCF role in the early years of 2000 were the changing healthcare climate and the fragmentation patients were experiencing with their care as a result of changing scheduling patterns of nurses, shorter lengths of stay, and the emergence of hospitalists. The PCFs *focus on the patients* in their 12-Bed Hospital, acting as that one nurse they can identify with during their hospitalization.

Metrics, generated by the PCF's geography on a patient unit, provided them constant feedback on their impact on quality measures, patient satisfaction, length of stay, and throughput (Figure 15-2). Through the use of *technology*, data specific to the individual PCF pinpointed their outcomes on a weekly basis. With a focused set of metrics, *outcomes* over time showed progressive *improvement* at Baptist Hospital (Robert Wood Johnson Foundation, 2007).

Beyond the 12-Bed Hospital

In 2007, the author had the opportunity to move to Washington, DC, where interest in the model of care from Baptist Hospital was high among the directors of nursing. As the author worked on many of the units at Washington Hospital Center as part of the introduction to the hospital, this was validated firsthand that care delivery was highly variable, as was the role of the nursing coordinator on each patient unit. The nursing coordinator was a quasi-management role designed to provide clinical expertise and management support on many of the patient units. In addition, after-hours nursing supervisors or coordinators, whose assignments were limited to a couple of departments, were also assigned to provide administrative and clinical support to nurses on the clinical units. Because of the scope of their assignments, both coordinators and supervisors had to prioritize which activities would be accomplished, and many had delegated management duties to assist the nurse managers in handling the workload. Advanced practice roles were also inconsistently assigned, some under nursing and others reporting to physician groups, and the APNs' alignment with the affairs of nursing was also variable. By realigning nursing support positions into management roles and clinical support roles, they were able to assign the required positions to pilot a model based on the 12-Bed Hospital model.

Figure 15-2 CNL Dashboard.

CLINICAL NURSE LEADER DASHBOARD

CORE MEASURES

GOAL	Jan	Feb	Mar	Apr	May	Jun	Jul	Aug	Sep	Oct	Nov	Dec
0 fallouts	0	0	0									

ACTION PLAN - CORE MEASURES | DATE
1 No core measure exceptions, continue to monitor
2
3

PATIENT FLOW - 11 AM & 2PM DISCHARGES

11:00 AM	Jan	Feb	Mar	Apr	May	Jun	Jul	Aug	Sep	Oct	Nov	Dec
GOAL 33%	6	11	6									

2:00 PM	Jan	Feb	Mar	Apr	May	Jun	Jul	Aug	Sep	Oct	Nov	Dec
GOAL 66%	33	37	35									

AVG. TIME 3:12 PM	Jan	Feb	Mar	Apr	May	Jun	Jul	Aug	Sep	Oct	Nov	Dec
	4:01	4:10	3:54									

ACTION PLAN - PT. THROUGHPUT | DATE
1 Encourage night staff to anticipate discharges
2 Frequent use of discharge board/checklist
3 Educate family on 11:00 AM discharge initiative

PERSONAL AND CLINICAL DEVELOPMENT PLAN

ACTION PLAN - DEVELOPMENT PLAN | DATE
1 Complete MSN by May 2010
2 Take CNL Certification Exam in July 2010
3 Learn APR-DRGs
4

PATIENT SATISFACTION - OVERALL

GOAL	Jan	Feb	Mar	Apr	May	Jun	Jul	Aug	Sep	Oct	Nov	Dec
90th Percentile	74.0	41.0	66.0	97.0								

ACTION PLAN -PATIENT SATISFACTION | DATE
1 Use scripting, encourage staff to be more consistent
2 Target new admissions and inform family on rounding process
3 Consistent walking rounds

LENGTH OF STAY (Top Three APR-DRGS)

1. APR-DRG 45 CVA & Cerebral Occlusion LOS - 8.7

GOAL 5.81	Jan	Feb	Mar	Apr	May	Jun	Jul	Aug	Sep	Oct	Nov	Dec
	8	11.2	10.2									

2. APR-DRG 47 TIA - LOS 3.0

GOAL 2.97	Jan	Feb	Mar	Apr	May	Jun	Jul	Aug	Sep	Oct	Nov	Dec
	2.5	3	2									

3. APR-DRG 53 Seizure - LOS 4.9

GOAL 3.72	Jan	Feb	Mar	Apr	May	Jun	Jul	Aug	Sep	Oct	Nov	Dec
	5.3	8.5	3.7									

ACTION PLAN - LENGTH OF STAY | DATE
1 Active participation on interdisciplinary LOS Stroke Meeting
2 Follow-up on stroke orders/ make sure all orders completed
3 Help expedite test results such as MRIs
4 Make sure all consults are called on time
5 Remind neurologist to expedite EEG reading
6 Manage family concerns about arrangements for post discharge
7
8
9

In this model, the creators chose a medical-surgical unit and identified baccalaureate-prepared staff members or coordinators interested in piloting this role. The group consulted with staff at the Baptist Hospital of Miami, and after an onsite visit they implemented the model on a pilot unit. The goal of this pilot was to evaluate key outcomes before and after implementation of the model, and use these data to further evaluate implementation on additional units.

The Clinical Nurse Leader Comes to Texas

In March of 2008, the author moved to the Dallas/Fort Worth area in Texas after being offered a system chief nurse role at Texas Health Resources (THR), a 14-hospital not-for-profit system in north Texas. A faith-based system with over 3,350 beds, 18,000 employees and 6,300 nurses, Texas Health was formed in 1997 by the merger of Presbyterian Health System, Harris Methodist Hospital System, and Arlington Memorial Hospital. Within the system are three Magnet-designated hospitals and six Pathways to Excellence–designated hospitals. Acute care hospitals within the system range from 36 to 866 licensed beds.

As the first system chief nurse, the author found unique nursing cultures and a common professional practice model based on the CPM Professional Practice Framework, nursing structures and processes, individualized to each setting. A Chief Nursing Officers Council (CNOC) had been in place for a number of years, and the chairperson role rotated annually among the CNOs within the system. One of the first activities was involving the CNOs in a strategic planning process that evaluated and prioritized key nursing and interdisciplinary strategies for the upcoming three years. Among the priorities identified was selecting and implementing a care model that acknowledges the changing climate within healthcare and addresses the future needs for care delivery in the hospitals.

The author was asked to review her work on the 12-Bed Hospital and educate the CNOs on the emerging role of the CNL. At that time (2008), the role of the CNL had not been implemented in any nongovernment healthcare facility in Texas. Consequently, the CNL curriculum had not been offered in any college in north Texas. At the strategic planning retreat, the CNOs determined that they would like to be the first system in Texas to implement the CNL role and they were also interested in modeling the care delivery model around the 12-Bed Hospital concept.

Considering the magnitude of this process, the CNOs determined that a pilot project would be needed to build a business case for a large-scale implementation.

Figure 15-3   Depiction of roles in three pathways of career development.

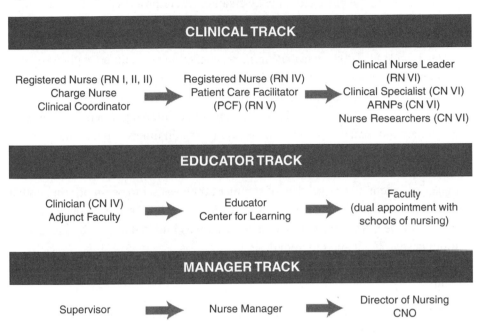

As the strategic plan was finalized, the nursing strategy involved the following components:

- Pilot the model on one medical-surgical unit in each Texas Health hospital in 2009.
- Study outcomes and results on the pilot units to determine extent of further development/implementation.
- Develop models that meet the needs of small, medium, and large hospitals.
- Provide an avenue for advancement of nursing staff professionally and educationally along a *clinical* career path while remaining at the bedside (see Figure 15-3).

In Figure 15-3, a fully defined path for clinical advancement is defined, building upon RN levels from 1 to 6. The educator and manager tracks were already well developed within the system. Clinical role progression had been much less defined and variable from one hospital to another. Through the addition of the patient care facilitator role at the baccalaureate level, and the CNL at the master's level, the career path would encourage nurse retention by creating career progression, and encourage nurses to advance into the CNL role, one that would allow nurses to advance, but remain at the bedside.

Harris and Ott (2008) state that "business cases must be built on explicit support action and strategically aligned anticipated outcomes that resonate throughout the organization and maintain strong partnerships with affiliating universities" (p. 25). As Texas Health CNOs contemplated a strategic educational partner, it was important that they choose a partner with the flexibility to gain timely support and approval from their universities for a CNL curriculum. The author approached leaders at the Texas Christian University in Fort Worth, Texas, and was greeted with interest and enthusiasm. A tentative target date of summer 2009 was set to begin offering both a generic CNL curriculum and a post-master's certificate, for advanced practice nurses interested in the CNL role. A development team was initiated to collaborate on curriculum development and program design.

The immediate deliverables determined for the pilot phase included the following:

- Determining the extent of further implementation and model configuration throughout the system
- Building a business case for the new model based on initial pilot outcomes
- Budgeting for further rollout of the model in 2010 and beyond
- Continuing to track and report outcomes
- Sharing the process and lessons learned from large-scale implementation of the CNL role in the private sector through publication/presentation

Determining Further Implementation and Model Configuration Throughout the System

In the strategic plan, a team was chartered to design a pilot of the PCF and CNL roles for every 12 to 16 beds on one medical-surgical unit across system hospitals ranging from 36 to 866 beds. To assist in that process, the Texas Health CNO leading the team used the tools available on the American Association of Colleges of Nursing Web site to formulate an implementation plan. Figure 15-4 details the first draft of the plan.

Figure 15-4 Texas Health Resources' initial implementation plan.

CNL Implementation Template for Texas Health Resources

Steps to Be Completed	Who Should Lead and Be Involved?	Why and How?
1. Organizational Culture		
A. Communicate the desired change to the CNL role.	**Lead:** System CNE and hospital CNOs	1. Add to system nursing strategic plan.
B. Make the case for change throughout the organization and hospitals.	**Lead:** System CNE and hospital CNOs **Involve:** Executive team, management and nursing staff, as well as physicians	2. Meet with system executive leadership and discuss. 3. Talk to hospital leadership including executive team, medical executive team, and nursing leadership.
C. Create an opportunity for clarity, discussion, dialogue, and learning.	**Lead:** CNOs, executive leadership, and nursing management	4. Offer forums for nursing staff to discuss concept.
2. Pre-implementation Work		
A. Select the right unit for implementation: responsive to change, leadership, and at-risk populations.	**Lead:** CNO, nursing directors **Involve:** Nursing leadership, CQO, potential CNLs	Create sample job descriptions, distribute for comment, and submit to corporate HR for evaluation and approval.
B. Create job descriptions: • BSN level • MSN level	**Lead:** CNO, HR	CNL role competencies, end-of-education program competencies, and competency checklists
C. Define the role of the CNL related to other clinical roles and functions that are present at the hospital and on the unit (CNS, case mgmt., etc.).	**Lead:** CNO, directors, educators, clinical support staff	Career ladder with defined CNL path
D. Consider the impact of the CNL on the clinical ladder.	**Lead:** CNO, directors, HR **Involve:** Clinical ladder team	Offer education sessions and bring system CNO to the meetings as appropriate.
E. Educate management on expectations of their role and leadership during the change process, how it should work, what they can do.	**Lead:** CEO/CNO **Involve:** Leadership team	Obtain corporate and hospital approval for additions to FTE budget.
F. Redesign the budget.	**Lead:** CNO **Involve:** Directors and managers	

Continues

Figure 15-4 Texas Health Resources' initial implementation plan (continued).

Steps to Be Completed	Who Should Lead and Be Involved?	Why and How?
3. Implementation		
A. Designate executive sponsor of the CNL implementation.	**Lead:** System CNE **Involve:** CNOs, hospital presidents	Secure buy-in and support of program.
B. Manager must support and champion the practice environment that maintains the integrity of the CNL role. (Manager operationalizes the role and the CNL actualizes it.)	**Lead:** Nursing directors **Involve:** Nurse managers and nursing supervisors	Create performance evaluation tool that focuses the CNL and nursing director and managers on successful outcomes or evidence of effective role implementation.
C. Embed the CNL role into the care delivery model. CNL to round daily with interdisciplinary team. CNL to communicate daily with all team members.	**Lead:** CNOs **Involve:** Nursing directors, nurse managers and supervisor, CNLs	
D. CNL and nursing director to meet 1–2 times per week to discuss challenges, successes, and continually to assist in evolving the role.	**Lead:** CNOs and nurse education	Focus on end-of-program competencies and required clinical experiences. What is the role at the individual facility?
E. Formal CNL orientation	**Lead:** CNO	
F. Ensure enculturation of the CNL role by meeting weekly/biweekly with the CNLs to accomplish the following: • Identify barriers and resolve barriers. • Identify successes and celebrate successes. • Communicate. • Provide support, leadership, and affirmation.	**Involve:** Nursing directors, nurse managers and supervisors, CNLs	
G. Create a process and format for tracking the implementation, with special attention given to noting incidences of success and challenging factors.	**Lead:** System CNE and CNOs **Involve:** Nursing directors and CNLs	
H. Communicate about the role and status at all major meetings (med exec, exec leadership, nursing leadership)	**Lead:** CNO/CQO/directors	

Figure 15-4 Texas Health Resources' initial implementation plan (continued).

Steps to Be Completed	Who Should Lead and Be Involved?	Why and How?
4. Outcomes		
A. Identify desired outcomes and evaluation model prior to implementation.	**Lead:** Joan Clark **Involve:** CNOs, nursing directors, quality staff	Review outcomes identified in CNL program proposal, and determine accuracy and application to the selected patient care setting.
B. Collect pre-implementation data that will be monitored post-implementation.	**Lead:** CNOs and nursing directors	

Building a Business Case for the New Model

In building a business case for implementation of a care model based around the CNL, the following was recommended:

- Gain buy-in from key stakeholders.
- Align program objectives with key quality, operational, and performance objectives.
- Provide justification for adding new FTEs (along with some reengineered roles).
- Align with unit management and other advanced practice roles.

The key to success will be the CNO's belief in the model and a passion for supporting the brave individuals who venture into the inaugural roles within the organization. To further develop each of these steps, consider the following.

Gain Buy-In From Key Stakeholders

The CNO can play a major role in defining and delineating the CNL role in concert with existing roles at the department level. An ideal method for building stakeholder support is to initiate a pilot of the model on a nursing unit where there is commitment and support from the managers and their direct reports, as well as passion for innovation and risk. With manager support, the individuals who venture into the pilot roles will act as ambassadors and role models of the proposed model. During the pilot phase, any and all feedback from key stakeholders should be amplified and acted upon in building ground-level support.

The CNO should also present progress and key results to a variety of audiences as part of a broader strategic initiative around promoting high-reliability patient care. Key audiences involved in building buy-in initially include the following:

- Senior executive team
- Hospital presidents
- Hospital chief quality officers
- System physician leadership committee
- System PI/patient safety steering committee
- System strategic planning committee: board of directors
- System quality committee: board of directors
- Boards of directors chairpersons
- Entity boards (selected)
- Nursing town halls/publications/entity practice councils

The use of visuals that will assist the CNO to effectively communicate how the role impacts other healthcare team members, patients and families, and physicians helps to prevent misconceptions about the role, such as "it's another layer of management" or "it's someone else who carries a clipboard and focuses only on one dimension of the care." See Figure 15-5 for a sample of a visual used at THR to describe the impact of the role to stakeholder groups.

Align Program Objectives With Key Quality, Operational, and Performance Objectives

Key outcomes are tracked before and after implementation to provide an accurate cost-benefit projection regarding important indicators such as reductions in avoidable events (e.g., pressure ulcers, DVT, falls), improvements in quality measures, patient throughput, and the like. Accurate accountings of these data are required, as well as a process for tracking progress before, during, and after pilot implementation. A strategy for projecting potential savings was devised based on a number of key indicators. See Figure 15-6 for an example. The method of calculation for each example indicator is explained in the following paragraphs.

In Figure 15-6, a report on current pressure ulcer incidence is generated for the unit selected to pilot the model. A projected level of improvement is indicated for the specific indicator as a result of CNL intervention. In estimating a projected improvement based on CNL intervention in the example related to pressure ulcers, an estimated 25% reduction is predicted, multiplied by the average cost per pressure ulcer

Figure 15-5   Visual aid to assist in presenting concepts to other stakeholders.

IMPACT OF THE CLINICAL NURSE LEADER ROLE

Physicians
- Diagnose and plan treatment
- Direct patient's plan of care
- Determine appropriate discharge plan
- Communicate with patient and family
- Collaborate with nursing and care team

APNs (CNS/ARNP)
- Is a clinical expert in assigned specialty/service line
- Consults on complex patient situations based on referrals from any of the members of the team
- Focuses on clinical care standardization around evidence-based practices for particular specialty or service line
- Collaborates with team in reviewing and revising care protocols

CNL
- Coordinates the care of clinical expert on assigned unit/beds (lateral integrator)
- All patients in assigned area
- Is able to distinguish between simple and complex case management requirements
- Keeps clinical staff informed of patients' progress to plan/is proactive in planning for patient needs (advocate)

- Case finds and coordinates d/c needs with social workers
- Consistently communicates plans between staff, physicians, and patients/families
- Designs, evaluates effectiveness of EBP guidelines and order sets in collaboration with medical staff and recommends changes as indicated
- Focused on quality, safety, and performance improvements at the microsystem level

RNs and Healthcare Team
- Provide and document plan of care
- Assist in developing and revising plan of care
- Communicate with patient, family, and other team members

Physicians

Clinical RNs and Other Care Team Members

Patient and Family

APNs

CNL

Medical Management Team

Documentation Specialist
- Reviews charts for core measures
- Reviews charts for "avoidable events"
- Reviews charts for POA

Social Worker
- Coordinates the discharge plan
- Is proactive in recognizing the potential for delay of d/c and has a backup plan
- Collaborates with the team, discusses d/c needs with physician, patient, and family
- Identifies psychosocial needs impacting discharge

Care Manager
- Communicates with all insurers and becomes proactive in defining LOS for each disease entity and reviews cases for optimum d/c potential
- Follows up on each denial, overturns on appeal
- Tracks denials by physician and by unit to identify trends, educates all involved parties

Figure 15-6 Representative example of metrics and goals for establishing cost-benefit of CNL implementation.

Metrics	42 AMH	THSH	4TTHHEB
1. Pressure ulcer reduction (based on 25%, @ $1,000/case)	$22,000	$8,250	$25,666
2. Fall reduction (based on 25%, @ $19,440/case)	$194,400	$41,222	$153,647
3. Core measures: • Pneumococcal vaccine • Discharge instructions	35	0	17
CHF (based on zero exceptions)	41	3	15
4. Patient satisfaction: • RNs kept me informed • Attention to special/personal needs • Adequate assistance for discharge (based on improvements from baseline)	73.9 74.4 73.3	82.7 83.0 71.1	81.3 84.0 80.0
5. Patient throughput: • % discharged by 11 am • % discharged by 2 pm	7.6% 17.4%	6.82% 37.08%	6.82% 37.08%

of $11,000, reported by the *Journal of the American Medical Association* in 2003. Similarly, a fall rate is calculated for the department and is based on a 25% reduction in falls at $19,440, as estimated in the work of Ann Hendrich (Hendrich, Nyhuis, Kippenbrock, & Soja, 2005).

Core measure exceptions are also tracked and reported for the pilot units. The expected target is zero exceptions for the pneumococcal vaccination of pneumonia patients and the documentation of discharge instructions with CHF patients. Targeted questions from the Press-Ganey patient satisfaction tool are monitored for the pilot units, and either an improvement from baseline or a specific target measure could be used to measure improvement. Finally, using a bed-tracking software package or reporting based on discharge time stamps in the hospital computer system, the percentage of patients discharged by 11:00 am and by 2:00 pm are tracked against benchmarks of 33% by 11:00 am and 66%, by 2:00 pm as a throughput efficiency measure.

H6THFW	7E-THD	5B-THP	M/STHW	3eTHK	MSTHC	Total
$22,000	$151,250	$46,750	$5,500	$11,000	$8200	$30,616
$302,320	$63,707	$101,182	$59,960	$33,727	$33,727	$985,872
25	16	1	15	16	2	
43	34	28	18	13	7	
81.8	87.9	78.0	88.0	82.3	81.4	
82.7	86.2	74.6	81.4	84.1	82.3	
81.1	78.8	73.8	80.9	74.8	79.9	
7.76%	6.82%	7.76%	6.82%	7.76%	6.82%	
27.4%	37.08%	27.4%	37.08%	27.4%	37.08%	

Although this is not an exhaustive list of measures that might be used in building a business case, the examples provide some representative ideas for how to build a template for measuring success with a CNL implementation. Figure 15-7 includes a more complete list of potential measures.

Depending on the type of department and the amount of opportunities specific to the specialty or the department's historical performance, it is also important to articulate specific objectives for improvement in advance of the pilot study, so that performance against the objectives can be monitored for improvements. Once the pilot is underway, it is also recommended that the CNLs themselves collect anecdotal evidence of their effectiveness, for example, something they may have caught regarding a specific patient under their care that, had it continued, would have complicated the patient's progress or added to a costly outcome of some kind. Those scenarios should be tracked and added to the overall cost-benefit analysis of the pilot implementation project. Also, it is recommended that a methodology be developed

Figure 15-7 Performance measures.

Quality Measures • Pneumonia vaccination • CHF discharge teaching Pay-for-Performance Documentation • Present on admission (POA) indicators Nurse-Sensitive Outcomes • Patient falls • Hospital-acquired pressure ulcers Prevention of Complications/Risk Avoidance • DVT • Nosocomial infections	Patient, Employee, and Physician Satisfaction Nursing Retention • First-year retention • Nurse vacancy Improved Patient Throughput • Average discharge time • 11 am and 2 pm discharge Cost Savings • Variable cost opportunities • LOS • Decreased overtime

for tracking individual CNL progress on expected outcomes for the patients specifically under their care. Those results should be regularly displayed on a scorecard or dashboard that is monitored and reviewed by the parties involved.

Provide Justification for Adding New FTEs

Whatever the model envisioned for implementing the CNL role, it often requires some creative approaches to justifying additional positions or looking to align other duties and positions within the hospital to accommodate a widespread implementation of the model. It really helped the author in Miami to have a CEO whose own objectives were also being addressed through the implementation of the 12-Bed Hospital model. The CEO supported the addition of FTEs needed to fully implement the model on all nursing units at Baptist. This meant that other nonnursing departments within the hospital were held back on adding volume-related positions over two budget years! Although this type of support may not be extremely realistic in today's economy and environment, the concept of recruiting an influential champion is advised, whether it is an important physician admitter, a board member who understands hospital operations, or the like. It helps to get help!

One might also plan a slow deployment of a hospital-wide model over a number of years. The longer the ramp-up time, the more time there is to build a solid business case for the continuation of the program. In my experience, after the pilot began at Baptist, word-of-mouth reports among the staff on other units about the pilot unit's successes made it unnecessary to sell the concept to staffs or physicians of other departments.

Another strategy is to justify the addition of positions by setting objective targets to reduce nursing costs such as overtime, the cost of new nurse turnover, use of contract labor, and so forth. The author recommends a conservative assumption, and continuous monitoring of results, so that the objectives are met. Once the assumptions around specific cost reductions come to pass in the outcomes, the results can be built into the prospective budgeting process to justify new positions.

Alignment With Unit Management and Other Advanced Practice Roles
Almost every model will have some unique roles and overlapping duties that can be realigned if a care delivery model around the role of the CNL is going to be widely implemented throughout the hospital or the system. In the author's experience at Miami, it was found that there were specific needs for the addition of ARNPs at night, available to the relatively high number of novice nurses assigned to that shift. We found their impact at night invaluable. So, when we began to ramp up the rapid response teams a few years ago, we added them to a 24-hour, 7-day coverage for the adult as well as the pediatric areas. These advanced practice nurses worked closely with the hospitalists, under their protocols, so they were able to assist them in coverage of their patients as well. The need for the clinical nurse specialist roles were examined, and the number of CNS positions were aligned with key strategic needs, such as specialists in wound and skin, pain and palliative care. Educator positions in the medical-surgical units and the medical-surgical specialties areas were pooled so these professionals could be used more efficiently to cover new staff. They were selected from the general pool of medical-surgical clinicians based on their areas of clinical expertise. This was done so that there could be a better match of skills with identified competency needs of new staff, based on assessment via the Performance Based Development System (PBDS).

Contemplating a multihospital implementation of the CNL role, it will be necessary to realign positions around consistent roles and leverage advanced practice and clinician roles across hospitals to regionalize support. In this way, the advanced practice staff can be truly a consultative resource to the CNLs at the front line. It will be necessary to be creative in aligning the roles so they can best assist hospitals, especially those who have not had the luxury of some of that support in the past. In this way, the alignment will also facilitate an alignment of the overall nursing service as well, which will serve us well with our strategic goal of pursuing eventual Magnet system designation.

As CNOs around the country continue to contemplate how they need to respond to some of today's realities in the healthcare system, as well as how they will respond to the future of patient care delivery, the work being done around the CNL role offers new hope.

Summary

- Texas Health strategies for multihospital implementation:
  - Use template for model development based on landmark work with the 12-Bed Hospital.
  - Use both a baccalaureate-prepared patient care facilitator (PCF) role, as well as the CNL role, to facilitate a pilot implementation that introduces a model of care delivery versus a singular role.
  - Pilot the model on one medical-surgical unit in each Texas Health hospital in 2009.
  - Study outcomes and results of the pilot program to determine extent of further development/implementation.
  - Look at effectiveness of model configuration in small, medium, and large hospitals.
  - Provide an avenue for advancement of nursing staff professionally and educationally along a *clinical* career path while remaining at the bedside.
- Pilot program deliverables:
  - Determine extent of further implementation and model configuration.
  - Build the business case for the new model based on initial pilot outcomes.
  - Budget for further rollout of model in 2010 and beyond.
  - Continue to track and report outcomes.
  - Share process and lessons learned from large-scale implementation of the CNL role in the private sector through publication/presentation.
- Building the business case for implementation within the context of a care delivery model can be difficult, especially if coupled with implementation in the context of a 12- to 16-bed assignment. Here are some suggested approaches:

- Gain buy-in from key stakeholders.
- Align program objectives with key quality, operational, and performance objectives.
- Provide justification for adding new FTEs (along with some reengineered roles).
- Align with unit management and other advanced practice roles.

Reflection Questions

1. Describe how the executive nurse administration leverages resources to increase capacity for the CNL role.
2. Identify strategies that guide executive administration in making the business case for the CNL.

Learning Activities

1. Review quality improvement data on one microsystem, outlining how these metrics might be improved with the implementation of a CNL.
2. Outline a dashboard for one clinical microsystem, and describe how the CNL would make a difference in improving outcomes.

Recommended Reading

Brown, C., Holcomb, L., Maloney, J., Naranjo, J., Gibson, C., & Russell, C. (2005). Caring in action: The patient care facilitator role. *International Journal of Human Caring, 9*(3), 51–58.

Weaver, D., & Sorrells-Jones, J. (2007, June). The business case as a strategic tool for change. *Journal of Nursing Administration, 37*(9), 414–420.

Wood, D. (2006, February). Twelve-bed hospital concept enhances patient care. *AMN Healthcare.* Retrieved April 3, 2009, from http://www.nursezone.com/nursing-news-events/more-features.aspx?ID=14753

References

American Association of Colleges of Nursing (AACN). (2007, February). *White paper on the education and role of the clinical nurse leader.* Retrieved on April 30, 2009, from http://www.aacn.nche.edu/Publications/WhitePapers/ClinicalNurseLeader07.pdf

Harris, J., & Ott, K. (2008, August). Building the business case for the clinical nurse leader role. *Nurse Leader, 6*(4), 25–28.

Hendrich, A., Nyhuis, A., Kippenbrock, T., & Soja, M. E. (2005). Hospital falls: Development of a predictive model for clinical practice. *Applied Nursing Research, 8*(3), 129–139.

Morjikian, R., Kimball, B., & Joynt, J. (2007, June). Leading change: The nurse executive's role in implementing new care delivery models. *Journal of Nursing Administration, 37*(9), 392–398.

Robert Wood Johnson Foundation. (2007, June). *12-Bed Hospital: Results*. Retrieved on April 30, 2009 from http://www.innovativecaremodels.com/care_models/10

Sherman, R., Shinkus Clark, J., & Maloney, J. (2008, June). Developing the clinical nurse leader role in the Twelve Bed Hospital model: An education/service partnership. *Nurse Leader, 6*(3), 54–58.

Shinkus Clark, J. (2004, May). An aging population with chronic disease compels new delivery systems focused on new structures and practices. *Nursing Administration Quarterly, 28*(2), 105–115.

APPENDIX A

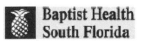 **Baptist Health South Florida**

Baptist Hospital of Miami
JOB DESCRIPTION

JOB TITLE: Patient Care Facilitator/Patient Care Facilitator, Advanced

DEPARTMENT: Patient Care
REPORTING RELATIONSHIP: Patient Care Center Manager
DATE ORIGINALLLY SUBMITTED: May 22, 2002
APPROVED BY: Vice President, Patient Care/Chief Nursing Officer

REVISED DATE: February 25, 2003

QUALIFICATIONS: The Patient Care Facilitator CN IV and Patient Care Facilitator Advanced is a level of the clinical tract to which a qualified applicant from outside Baptist Hospital may apply without completing prior levels on the Professional Nursing Advancement Program. This level recognizes broad clinical and educational expertise and regularly 24-hour/7-day accountability.

Patient Care Facilitator Educational/Experiential Requirements

- Baccalaureate degree in nursing or working towards degree; Three years acute care experience, in clinical specialty, within the last two years.
- Documentation of Florida Registered Nurse Licensure.
- Certification preferred in the clinical specialty area.
- Validation of CPR instructor and/or ACLS/PALS/NALS certification.
- Documentation of the continuing education requirements for the CNIV (32 hours over the last year), with a minimum of 6 in leadership.
- Validation of active participation and/or leadership in a unit base committee.
- Clinical maturity and expertise.
- Excellent interpersonal skills.
- Collaboration and negotiation skills.
- Knowledge of managed care and reimbursement principles.

- Proficiency in the nursing process, problem solving and the performance improvement process.
- Capability of priority setting.
- Effective oral and written communication skills.
- Team building skills.
- All applicants are committed to a minimum of modified full time employment. The scheduling of the tour of duty must remain flexible to meet the changing needs of the clinical service and the patient caseload.

Patient Care Facilitator Advanced
In addition to the above the Patient Care Facilitator Advanced will have:
- BSN with MSN or MS in a health care related field or matriculating towards either Masters degree within 2 years.
- Certification in the clinical specialty area or obtain within one year.
- Skill in defining and observing clinical competencies and required synergies for a unit base patient population.
- Demonstrated leadership as a change agent in an interdisciplinary team responsible for clinical outcomes.
- Skill in mentoring colleagues and other Patient Care Facilitators.

JOB SUMMARY/PURPOSE:

Patient Care Facilitator
- Is an advanced Clinical Nurse who leads the practice of nursing and manages care on the unit.
- Is recognized as being proficient in the delivery of complex nursing care.
- Continuously promotes quality patient care by coordinating patient care conferences; Assists in the development and revision of pathways.
- Assumes a broad level of accountability for the outcomes of care for a select population of patients throughout their stay on a designated unit

Patient Care Facilitator Advanced
- In addition to the above the Patient Care Facilitator Advanced:
- Seeks out learning opportunities for the unit staff and serves as an expert resource for all aspects of nursing care delivery.
- Works closely with the Leadership Team in planning clinical goals and objectives.
- Is responsible for data collection and analysis, variance identification and extrapolation, establishment of reporting mechanisms, communication methodologies, care giver adherence to program objectives and ultimately, evidencing quality care in a defined period of time.
- Is certified in the clinical specialty area.

PSYCHOLOGICAL CONSIDERATIONS:

Able to work under stressful situations and respond to emergencies competently. Able to work as a part of an Interdisciplinary team. Must be flexible, have problem solving skills, prioritize and demonstrate healthy coping mechanism

ENVIRONMENTAL CONSIDERATIONS:

Potential contamination/exposure to bloodborne pathogens, body substances, biohazardous materials and infectious diseases. Able to work in a temperature controlled hospital environment, occasional exposure to a variety of auditory and olfactory stimuli.

ESSENTIAL JOB FUNCTIONS:

Assessment

1. Obtains baseline information utilized for the development of individualized patient plan of care
2. Conducts patient rounds on current caseload, evaluating goals with physician or interdisciplinary team.
3. Monitors patient's progress against plan of care until discharge from designated patient care area.
4. Collaborates with interdisciplinary team members to identify potential barriers and variances to the plan of care.

Planning

1. Coordinates the plan of care with patients, family and interdisciplinary team.
2. Plans discharge needs beginning at the time of admission.
3. Assists with the development of protocols/standards/pathways.
4. Leads interdisciplinary team meetings and rounds.
5. Promotes development of clinical practice based on research and evidence.
6. Assists leadership team with maintenance of initial and ongoing unit-based clinical competencies.

Implementation

1. Acts as a liaison between patients, caregivers and community resources.
2. Educates interdisciplinary team, patient/family on plan of care.
3. Serves as a direct care provider, as appropriate, to ensure outcome obtainment.
4. Provides patient/family teaching using available resources and tools.
5. Uses and individualizes disease specific pathways to obtain patient goals.
6. Implements strategies to reduce resource consumption and length of stay for assigned patients.
7. Educates patients, families and interdisciplinary team on the Care Manager role.
8. Acts as consultant to clinical staff in assisting with unfamiliar procedures/treatments.
9. Assists with presenting results, trends or conclusions from analysis of patient's outcomes to patient focused committees.

10. Utilizes process of performance improvement.
11. Promotes patient safety.
12. Communicates changes in plan of care to the patient/family and the health care team members in a timely manner.
13. Demonstrates creativity and innovation in approach to complex problem solving.
14. Leads crisis management
15. Acts as a change agent.
16. Provides coverage to other Patient Care Facilitators and directs care providers as appropriate to ensure outcome obtainment.
17. Delegates aspects of care to qualified personnel.
18. Promotes quality patient care by coordinating patient care conferences.

Evaluation
1. Evaluates plan of care and makes revisions based on condition changes and variances.
2. Evaluates patient progress towards expected outcomes.
3. Evaluates staff competencies and reports to leadership team.
4. Assist in the comparison of available data at the local/State/National level.
5. Participates in staff evaluations

Professional Accountability
1. Coordinates and delegates pilot studies for product review and/or care delivery.
2. Attends Clinical Practice Council meetings as needed.
3. Acts as role model and demonstrates expertise in conflict resolution and negotiation.
4. Participates in unit collaborative committees.
5. Develops and maintains clinical expertise in the care of a designated patient population.
6. Demonstrates professional independence in the practice of nursing.
7. Consults internal experts when appropriate.
8. Attends 75% and/or assumes a leadership role in a unit base committee.
9. Maintains documentation of the continuing education requirements for the CNIV (32 hours over the last year) with a minimum of 6 in leadership.
10. Participates in at least one community health and/or teaching project per year.
11. Maintains certification in the clinical specialty area.
12. Maintains CPR instructorship; ACLS, PALS, or NALS provider card.
13. Promotes the development of staff registered nurses, through the professional nursing advancement program.

Leadership
1. Leads the team to achieve patient outcomes.
2. Selects and develops team members.
3. Monitors and evaluates staff and the team's clinical outcomes.
4. Develops an individual leadership plan and meets objectives

Addendum
PATIENT CARE FACILITATOR ADVANCED

1. Assumes a leadership role in practice team meetings and facilities productive working relationships among members.
2. Promotes development of clinical practice based on research and evidence.
3. Assists with the development and maintains a unit-based competency system in collaboration with the leadership team.
4. Develops and coordinates protocols/standard orders/pathways.
5. Incorporates findings or variance analysis in the unit and/or organization-wide performance improvement.
6. Attends 75% and/or assumes a leadership role in a hospital committee.
7. Documents continuing education for the CN IV (36 hours over the last year) with a minimum of 6 hours in leadership.
8. Maintains membership in a professional organization. Seeks out learning opportunities for the staff.
9. Serves as an expert resource for all aspects of nursing.
10. Works closely with the leadership team in planning clinical goals and objectives.
11. Assists with presentations of trends or conclusions, for analysis of patient outcomes, to patient focused committees.
12. Functions as an expert for all aspects of nursing care delivery.
13. Assumes responsibility for mentoring and for staff development on the assigned unit.
14. Participates in the development of staff hospital-wide.
15. Shares accountability for unit-based and hospital-wide performance improvement through interdisciplinary committees.

ADA CRITERIA:

Standing	To set up equipment, too deliver direct care, to informally discuss issues with members of health team, to teach.
Sitting	To educate, teach, counsel patients/families, to conduct/attend meetings, to facilitate/participate in multidisciplinary team conference
Walking	To move about units and between units for rounds, to visit/assess patients to deliver direct patient care
Pushing/Pulling	To move audiovisual equipment, to deliver direct patient care.
Squatting/Kneeling	To provide CPR, to deliver direct patient care.
Lifting	To move audiovisual equipment, to provide direct patient care.
Vision	To read charts, to use audiovisual aids, to assess patients/families/environments.
Hearing	To assess patients/families/environments, to listen to verbal information from patient/families/health care teams.
Speaking	To communicate with others in English.

AGE SPECIFIC CRITERIA (check appropriate ages)		DEMONSTRATED COMPETENCY
	Neonate	
	Infant	
	Child	
	Adult	
	Geriatric	

SIXTEEN

Best Practices from Clinical Nurse Leaders

■ James L. Harris

■ **Learning Objectives**

- Analyze best practices of CNLs across practice settings.
- Discuss the importance of the CNL/ nurse manager partnership.

"Realize your influence and use it wisely ... inspire people to excel while things are happening at lightning speed."

Captain Michael Abrashoff

Key Terms

Partnership

Safety

Change

Exemplars

Evidence-based practice

Impact

Outcomes improvement

Innovation

Quality

CNL Roles

Outcome manager

Systems analysis/risk anticipator

Clinician

Client advocate

Educator

Information manager

CNL Professional Values

Accountability

Integrity

CNL Core Competencies

Communication

Designer/manager/coordinator
  of care

Provider and manager of care

Illness and disease management

Nursing technology and resource
  management

Introduction

As Lily Tomlin once stated, "I always wondered why somebody didn't do something about that. Then I realized I was somebody." This statement has a familiar ring when one considers the partnership that was created by academic institutions and practice settings in response to quality, effective, and safe care demands. The partnership culminated with the introduction of the clinical nurse leader (CNL) role, an advanced nurse generalist educated at the master's degree level who practices within the microsystem. Since the introduction of the role in 2004, many academic institutions have prepared CNLs and practice settings are including the role in staff allocations. The early CNL pioneers have many documented successes, and the impact of their actions is evident in practice settings across the continuum of care. Exemplars of CNLs were gleaned from presentations at a 2009 CNL Clinical Summit and are spotlighted in one of the following domains: quality and safety, financial considerations, and satisfaction and innovation.

Quality and Safety

Improving Patient Education on an Inpatient Psychiatric Unit Utilizing the Plan-Do-Study-Act Model

Suzanne VanBoening

Documentation of patient education was inconsistent and vague upon review of medical records for patients admitted to an inpatient psychiatric unit. This led to an intervention aimed at improving patient education documentation in three areas: diagnosis, medications, and coping skills. The CNL initially calculated current compliance and collaborated with information technology specialists. Together we created a "patient education deficit" problem field with 30 interventions for registered nurses (RNs) to select when entering computerized entries. Education prior to implementation was provided. Pre- and postintervention data revealed the following positive outcomes by domain.

Diagnosis

Target: 75%
Precompliance: 5% to postcompliance: 88% (average)

Medication Education

Target: 75%
Precompliance: 0% to postcompliance: 83% (average)

Crisis Planning

Target: 75%
Precompliance: 5% to postcompliance: 57% (average)

Clinical Nurse Leader Impact on Veterans Administration Inpatient Admission Assessment

Mary T. Dellario, Ellen M. Asbury, and Robyn Mitchell

Although a computerized medical record is advantageous for data retrieval, timely and complete entries can be challenging. Incomplete and untimely entries result in decreased intra- and interdisciplinary communication and handoffs from shift to shift. Clinical nurse leaders assigned to inpatient care units collectively developed a systematic method for timely and accurate completion of initial assessments, resulting in a 91% compliance rate from an 81% rate, thus expediting discharge planning, interdisciplinary communication, handoffs, and reduced length of stay. Phase II of the strategy is planned and will focus on evaluating the impact of CNL activities measured in terms of quality and safe patient outcomes.

Respiratory Failure: Can We See It Coming?

Carrie Tierney

Concerned with the number of readmissions to critical care units secondary to respiratory decompensation, a CNL assessed the impact of a process improvement strategy aimed at improving respiratory deterioration identification and reducing frequency of codes, the number of intubations, and the number of deaths related to unidentified respiratory decompensation. Through a series of staff education and patient assessments many successful outcomes have resulted including decreased readmissions, interventions with patients that reduced respiratory complications, and opportunities for novice nurses to enhance skills and critical thinking abilities.

The CNL Role: Face It, Understand It, and Showcase It

Connie Shipley, Shannon Kartchner, Diane L. Kelly, and George E. Wahlen

During periods of turmoil, instability, and change within the microsystem, the CNL can serve a vital role in maintaining quality of care and effecting positive change. Introducing the CNL role in units in which the turnover rate for nurse leaders and staff are high and no earmarked funding for the role existed, the CNL can face challenges from the beginning. Pivotal to success is the development of a strong partnership among the CNL, academic partner, and the nurse manager. The CNL is the transformational clinical leader who builds a foundation for vertical and lateral leadership teams to change the practice environment and shift power to staff and patients. This proved successful on an acute medicine unit resulting in a strong partnership, reduced staff turnover, and quality outcomes such as reduction in restraint use, pressure ulcers, and falls.

The CNL Role in Nontraditional Settings: Emergency Department

Jennifer A. Jones

The traditional CNL role has primarily been described as leading a small cohort of patients in a hospital unit. However, in a highly complex emergency department (ED), over 200 patients daily may receive treatment. A CNL assigned to an ED focused on evidence-based clinical quality improvement of micropopulations. The improvement began with a unit analysis for falls risk. Findings revealed increased numbers of falls among patients who entered the ED for treatment who were intoxicated and more likely to be a suicide risk, subsequently requiring the use of restraints after a fall. The CNL developed and educated staff on falls precautions, reduction in use of restraints, and use of a suicide assessment tool. "Real-time patient reviews" were used in order to transition evidence into practice. Emergency department falls were reduced by 98% and the time spent in restraints by 24%. Additionally, 100% of patients who required 1:1 suicide observation, as scored by the assessment tool, were placed in the correct safety watch, an intervention previously missed by ED staff. Following these sustained successful interventions, the CNL has initiated other evidence-based practices that focus on chest pain/acute myocardial infarction and door-to-balloon time from ED arrival to the cardiac catheterization suite.

Clinical Nurse Leaders "Bridge Quality"

Mary De Ritter and Kathy Faber

The CNL is an instrument for transforming nursing to an evidence-based practice environment. Two CNLs practicing in different neonatal intensive care units implemented evidence-based activities that improved discharge processes. The interventions focused on providing staff with current information and practices. Team building was enhanced, activities by staff were coordinated that reduced duplication, and the discharge process was a satisfying experience for staff and families. Using evidence to guide practice, learning, improvement processes, and equitable resource management occur, as evidenced in the two different units and separate medical centers.

The Clinical Nurse Leader and Nurse Manager Partnership

Judd E. Strauss and Mary Jo Loughlin

A key indicator of success for the CNL role is the establishment of a partnership with the unit nurse manager from the outset. From the decision to employ a CNL, the partnership emerged that included the delineation of role and functions of the CNL, nurse manager, and staff. This action was recognized as a primacy factor influencing the success and impacts of the CNL. The CNL is recognized as the clinical staff member who engages in risk assessments; developing interventions that focus on safety, quality, positive work environments, and interdisciplinary communication; the link between the patient, staff, and multiple physician specialties; and the forces driving evidence-based practice. National benchmarks are maintained, satisfaction scores are high, and staff morale remains positive. The CNL is the primary catalyst for the positive outcomes.

The Clinical Nurse Leader and the Clinical Nurse Specialist: Complementary Roles Resulting in a Wider Platform From Which to Strengthen Patient Care and Nursing Practice

Lynne A. Ludeman and Jennifer Spiker

From its inception, the CNL role has been accompanied by confusion, particularly with respect to the difference between the CNL and the clinical nurse specialist (CNS). To address this concern, a synergistic interplay between the two roles was approached by differentiating the roles as complementary approaches: the CNL as microsystem and the CNS as macrosystem. The CNL, well versed as a generalist in the needs of a unit, can strengthen the role of the CNS, a hospital-wide specialist. This complementary approach was realized when the need to reduce urinary tract infection (UTI) rates was addressed during the Magnet journey. By approaching this patient care issue from two different vantage points, the synergy of the CNL and CNS expanded the breadth of practice and UTI rates were reduced.

Clinical Nurse Leaders: Enhancing Performance Improvement and Closing the Gap in Nursing Documentation

Sara Gravelle and Amanda Brown

Clinical nurse leaders added a new dimension to a performance improvement initiative, the reduction of peripheral intravenous (IV) infiltrations. Risk management assessment of current nursing documentation practices revealed gaps in information about how IV infiltration occurred in the facility, the severity, and nursing interventions upon discovery of an infiltrate. The CNLs collaborated with clinical effectiveness in developing a supplemental documentation tool to improve consistency of peripheral IV assessment. An evidence-based infiltration scale was used to grade infiltrates, and nurses were educated to follow a cluster of interventions based in the grade of infiltrate. The tool was used hourly at the bedside to document assessment of five site characteristics and visibility. Additionally, the tool was used to collect data related to IV infiltrates and actions taken following the infiltrate. This patient-centric performance improvement initiative required commitment and perseverance, and impacts of practice of the point of care remain constant.

The Adult Tracheostomy Team

Nicole Manchester, Micheline Chipman, Davide Ciraculo, Jean Fecteau, Sonja Orff Ney, Darlene Rouleau, Dabuekke Tabor, and Joel McMullin
A quality improvement project was initiated to address the variation in care and management of the adult patient with a tracheostomy. A strategy to use and promote evidence-based practice and standardized care followed, focusing on minimizing complications. Using a microsystems approach, an interdisciplinary team examined what resources were needed and available, the supply chain, and care at the bedside for the adult patient with a tracheostomy. A database was created to identify and begin setting team goals for various points of care and metrics. Preliminary results reveal care improvements and increased communication among all care providers. These were enhanced by rounds and standardization of care at the beside.

Improving Breastfeeding Outcomes by Implementation of Evidence-Based Practice on a Postpartum Unit

Anjanetta Davis

Despite the many documented benefits of breastfeeding, only a small percentage of new mothers at one healthcare facility were breastfeeding, less than half the established benchmark (71%/33%). The low rate was compounded by findings of increased supplemental feedings, lack of staff involvement, and inadequate documentation. Several interventions followed, including revision of the breastfeeding policy, nursery standing order review, changes in the flow sheet, staff education, and patient education. Outcomes evidence postimplementation breastfeeding rates increased from 16% to 31%, the supplementation rate decreased from 71% to 66%, and breastfeeding documentation during each shift increased.

Patient Safety Through Effective Communication During Disaster Relief

Mary E. Mather

To improve patient safety through accurate communication among nurses, physicians, and emergency medical technicians during disaster relief, a standardized method for clinical handoffs during transition of evacuees to a shelter occurred. The handoff strategy was implemented to improve communication among providers and emergency medical technicians. The HUDDLE strategy (team members in a huddle as a group) was used to come together and discuss a plan. Improved patient satisfaction, communication among all personnel, and accuracy in delivery of care were the outcomes.

Know the Game Plan: HUDDLE

Kim Hall

Failures in communication among healthcare teams result in detrimental patient health outcomes, appointment inaccessibility, and patient dissatisfaction. The CNL is central to interventions that can reduce these. A geriatric evaluation and management (GEM) clinic staff identified that fragmented communication resulted in multiple missed patient opportunities. Following education on access and team communication, a new process (HUDDLE) emerged before morning and afternoon clinics that focused on discussions regarding appointment availability and critical patient issues. Since implementing the collaborative HUDDLE, higher clinic utilization rates, higher capacity, enhanced situation monitoring, communication among staff, and higher patient satisfaction has occurred.

Microsystem Best Practices: The Role of the CNL With Improving Medication Compliance

Darlene Rouleau

The inability for patients to follow prescribed medication regimens adversely effects patient outcomes. An intervention proven to have several benefits, including improved medication adherence, is postdischarge follow-up phone calls. A CNL conducted a survey to assess the current process for patient follow-up phone calls. This resulted in a list of the inpatient units that conducted follow-up calls and the common language or scripts used by staff. Using this information, a structured and standardized approach is planned for implementation throughout the facility, including standardized record keeping. The impact of the CNL's actions at the microsystem level has implications for the macrosystem.

Clinical Nurse Leaders Influencing Systems Change: Influenza and Pneumococcal Vaccinations

Christina Hericks, Lisa Hubbard, and Jillian Jacob

It is recommended that patients with high-risk diagnoses receive vaccinations for influenza and pneumococcal disease. An innovative plan was developed and executed by CNLs at one facility that resulted in a significant increase in vaccinations. The increase required a series of actions to accomplish the goal: (1) reviewing the current system of documenting vaccinations; (2) changing the electronic processes for screening, ordering, and documentation; and (3) adopting new processes that allowed nurses to order and administer vaccinations based on approved protocols. This is one example of how CNLs can have a significant impact that is need based.

AONE Transitioning Care at the Bedside (TCAB) Proposal

Rebecca Pomrenke and Stephanie S. Brown

Transitioning care at the bedside is one initiative that continues to impact the delivery of safe and quality care. A participating facility in the TCAB project has taken nursing hourly rounds to a new height, resulting in improved care, recognition for the rounds, and enhanced patient satisfaction. During rounds, nurses initiated a checklist that provided visual questions to check: the "5 Ps" (pain, potty, position, possessions, and pumps). As a secondary aim, reduction in the number of call lights was desired. Prior to and following this intervention, the total numbers of call lights were tracked. Preliminary outcomes evidence a reduction in the number of call lights from 148 to 83 on the day shift and an increase in patient satisfaction from 4.57 to 4.83. These outcomes support the notion that nursing rounds are a value-added activity in which staff address needs and increase purposeful contact with patients. Numerous other anecdotal findings are a result of the intervention and are being documented.

Educational Program for Patients With Congestive Heart Failure

Karen Bennett and Suzanne Brown

The rate of hospitalized patients with congestive heart failure (CHF) has steadily increased. Two CNLs developed a CHF educational program using a cost-effective and proven tool, a loose-leaf booklet provided to patients at admission and used by staff to reinforce care goals. To evaluate the outcomes of this action, a patient questionnaire was developed for completion before discharge and follow-up calls by the CNL are planned to continuously evaluate the educational impact. Readmission rates will also be tracked as a quality and financial indicator.

Financial Considerations

A Clinical Nurse Leader's Use of Evidence-Based Practice in the Reduction of PICC Line

Tammy Lee

The increasing rise of hospital-acquired infections resulted in national incentives by the Institute of Medicine, Institute for Healthcare Improvement, and The Joint Commission. Simultaneously, pay for performance reimbursement methodology required providers to address the national initiatives. A review of performance improvement data revealed an increase in PICC line infections from the previous year. This resulted in an evidence-based intervention in which a new protocol, a customized dressing change kit, was approved, and a new nursing care plan format was adopted. Cost of the initiative to reduce bloodstream infections, including PICC line infections, was $14.00 per patient. The savings netted $500,000. A year following the intervention, a 50% reduction in PICC line–associated bloodstream infections was attained.

Implementing a Change Process to Expand the CNL Program

Charlotte J. Birkenfeld, Christine Cobb, and Lisa Maree

Using action research methodology, CNLs and nurse managers crafted a business plan in order to expand the number of CNLs within a healthcare facility. A four-prong approach was used as supporting documentation for the plan: (1) the early years of the CNL program, (2) taking stock of CNL accomplishments, (3) a new beginning, and (4) CNL role implementation and expansion throughout the facility. The primary driver of the business plan was the impact metrics of practicing CNLs and the projected impact of additional positions across the continuum of care. To date, the impact of existing CNLs evidence reduction in falls and pressure ulcers, increased patient satisfaction, and improved and accurate nursing documentation. When one considers the financial metrics associated with a fall with injury and a hospital-acquired pressure ulcer, the annual salary of a CNL can easily be justified, as can the addition of further positions.

Utilization of the Clinical Nurse Leader in a Health Department Setting

Patricia Egan

In a health department system in which no job classification exists for a CNL, creativity is essential to role implementation. Role implementation progressed through a series of discussions with nursing leadership regarding the benefits of the position and the unique skill set possessed by a CNL. What followed was the incorporation of the role into the senior community health nursing supervisor's position. Because of the inconsistencies in clerical procedures, process mapping, and procedure development for areas such as appointments, the CNL initiated a project for check-in and cashier. By standardizing these processes, the organization has been able to improve orientation and training of employees and has decreased the error rate, which directly affects billing. Other projects initiated by the CNL included improving the physical layout of the clinic, thereby reducing wait time in the physician's clinic, thus increasing patient satisfaction and access to prenatal care. Successes have resulted in peers and administrators valuing the role, and it is hoped that CNLs will continue to expand and develop to a regional level and eventually statewide.

The CNL Immersion Experience When You're the Only One

Terri Gaiser

The CNL immersion experience is designed to allow for a "real-world," practical experience that will be needed to be successful in practice. This becomes a challenge when you are the first and only CNL in the area. My immersion was a partnership between the university, the medical center's director of nursing, and myself. Projects were designed that allowed demonstration of the impact of the role by improving outcomes. The experience was adapted to fit the organizational needs by addressing problems in several different departments, each with specific microsystem needs and goals. The nursing director provided guidance and support within the organization, and the university ensured that I was working within the CNL role. Regular meetings occurred to monitor progress and discuss issues. One of the outcomes improved in the CNL immersion involved central lines. Central line sites were evaluated and discussions with key players followed. Strategies were developed to reduce central line infections, thus resulting in significant savings and positive patient outcomes.

A CNL Student Capstone Project: Abdominal Pain Protocol and Shorter Stay in an Emergency Department

Janie Decker

There has been a steady increase in emergency department (ED) visits, contributing to overcrowding and increased length of stay in an era of decreased inpatient beds and reimbursement. Compounding the issues is the number of patients presenting to EDs with abdominal pain, 5% to 10% of visits. A CNL capstone project focused on implementation of evidence-based care and use of best practices to design care of ED patients experiencing abdominal pain. A series of interactions and education with staff on using evidence-based order sets were required, resulting in improved patient outcomes and a redesigned care delivery system, demonstrating more efficient and cost effective care. Key players included CNLs, discharge coordinators, and social workers. Following a workshop focusing on coordination of care and discharge planning, a clinical care coordination team was formed that included delineation of role and functions, thus enhancing discharge processes. The CNL was the placement coordinator for patients, from the acute to skilled setting, and collaborated with the social worker, staff, and discharge coordinator. The success has been measured in decreased length of acute stays and coordinated transfer to skilled settings. This is one of many approaches the CNL can initiate and function as a team coach toward a desired goal.

Satisfaction and Innovation

Improving Inpatient Satisfaction Scores: One CNL's Initiative

Laurel B. Scaff

Patient satisfaction has stepped into the limelight as an important indicator of quality of care. Thus, it has become of utmost importance that healthcare institutions take time to survey patients and use the data to identify areas for improvement. The CNL seized the opportunity to be innovative and create two initiatives that would potentially have a positive impact on patient satisfaction scores. The initiatives included a postdischarge call and scripting for the CNL to use daily during rounds with patients and families. This was made possible by networking with other facilities to obtain best practices for postdischarge calls and scripting for daily rounds. As a result of the initiative, satisfaction has steadily increased, creating success for patients and staff providing care.

Integration of the Clinical Nurse Leader With the Development of a Pediatric Progressive Care Unit

Denise Walker

Assessment of neonatal and pediatric intensive care units revealed a number of patients who have progressed from a life-threatening state to a medically stable condition. Many patients' stay in the intensive care units is restrictively mandated only by nursing hours required for care. Progressive care units, which offer an increase in nursing hours to medically stable patients, are emerging as a viable alternative for this population. Favorable outcomes include decreased cost, increased satisfaction, and support for the concept of a pediatric progressive care unit (PPCU). Recognizing the positive potential for a PPCU, a CNL role was included in the staffing for the unit. The role was targeted to be the liaison: the CNL assesses patients in the pediatric intensive care unit and the neonatal intensive care unit for potential transfer to the PPCU. The success of the role was not without growing pains, but over time, ranking of the facility on confidence and trust in nurses have increased. This innovation is another example of the value of the CNL role at the microsystem level.

The Impact of Clinical Nurse Leader and Nurse Manager Partnership on Patient Care

Michelle Carpentier and Angela M. Creta

The vision of implementation was a partnership between the CNL and unit nurse manager that would positively impact patient outcomes, improve collaboration, and increase utilization of evidence-based nursing. The delineation of roles of the CNL and nurse manager has been the key to success. As a result of this partnership, pressure ulcers have decreased, communication among staff and providers has increased, and actions are being based on evidence including the development of clinical guidelines. The nurse manager is able to dedicate the time necessary for effectively managing the unit while the CNL manages care processes.

The Clinical Nurse Leader Association (CNLA)

Mary Stachowiak

As the CNL role has been introduced throughout the United States in a variety of healthcare facilities, a group of CNLs decided to be proactive and develop an association aimed at (1) creating a sustainable organization to support and promote CNLs and their contributions; (2) creating relevant forums for CNLs to collaborate, network, and celebrate contributions; (3) ensuring evidence-based practice and innovation is fostered by CNLs; and (4) establishing critical relationships with interested stakeholders who can anchor the CNL as the recognized integrator of quality and safety at the point of care. The inaugural officers are Mary Stachowiak, president; Nina Swan, vice president; Tammy Lee, secretary; and Kim Murray, treasurer. Board members include Marge Wiggins, practice partner; Jane Gannon, educator; Joan M. Stanley, AACN member; Paula Miller, VA board representative; and Beth Aronson, administrative assistant. It is such innovative and creative actions by this group of CNLs and others that validate the future of the association and the ongoing realization of how those in the role will be transformers of health care.

INDEX

A

AACN. *See* American Association of Colleges of Nursing

Abrashoff, Michael, 287

academic partnerships, 21–61
American Association of Colleges of Nursing, 25
defining partnership, 25
examples, 28–30
gap analysis, 27
partnership formation process, 29
Robert Wood Johnson Foundation, 25
sustaining of partnerships, 31
University of Maryland Medical Center, 28–30
Vanderbilt University School of Nursing, 30
Veterans Affairs Medical Centers of Tennessee Valley Healthcare System, 15, 30, 40

academic preparation, 227–238

academic programs, 221–241
clinical preparation, 227–238
collaboration, 235
communication, 234
course titles/examples, 238
curricular models, 225–227
dignity, 233
education tools, 239
information sharing, 235
needs assessment, 228
outcomes management project, 229
quality outcomes management, 231
relationship building, 234
respect, 233
safety, 231
socialization, 223–224
workflow, 236

acceptance, 87–88

access to health care, 202

accountability, 89

active listening, 96

acute myocardial infarction, 14

"The Adult Tracheostomy Team," 294

advanced practice registered nursing, 10

advisory council, 45–61
charter, 50
collaboration, 46–60
conduct meeting, 53
draft charter, 49